PLANNING A

DETOX

BECCA THOMAS

Published in 2002 by Caxton Editions
20 Bloomsbury Street
London WC1B 3JH
a member of the Caxton Publishing Group

© 2002 Caxton Publishing Group

Designed and produced for Caxton Editions
by Open Door Limited
Rutland, United Kingdom

Editing: Mary Morton
Setting: Richard Booth
Digital imagery © copyright 2002 PhotoDisc Inc.

Title: **Planning a Detox**
ISBN: 1 84067 286 2

PLANNING A

DETOX

BECCA THOMAS

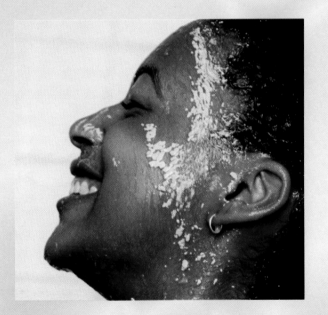

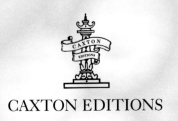

CAXTON EDITIONS

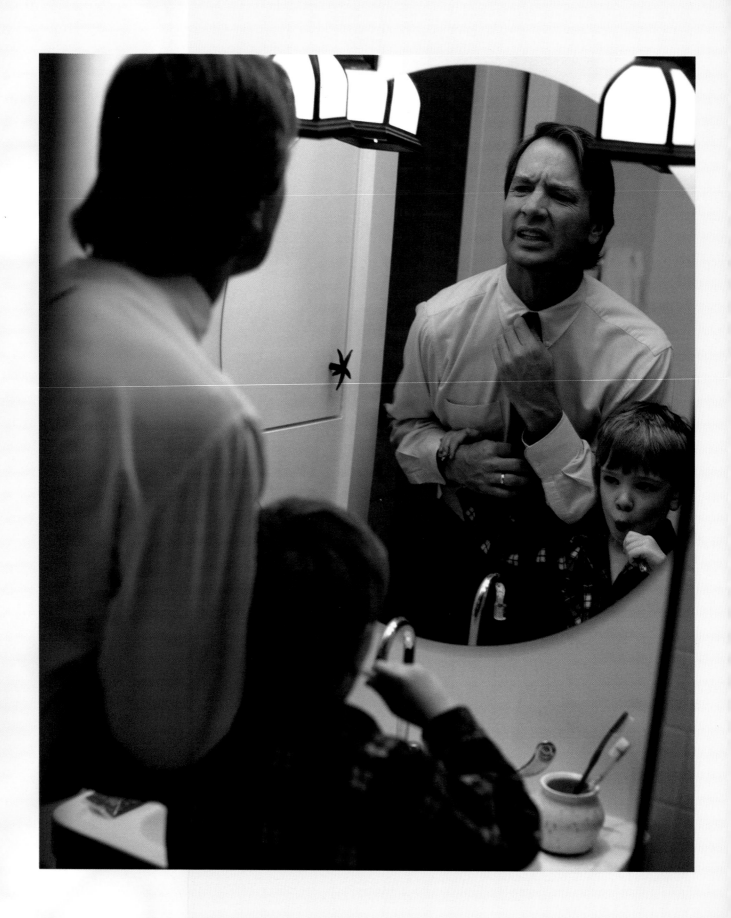

CONTENTS

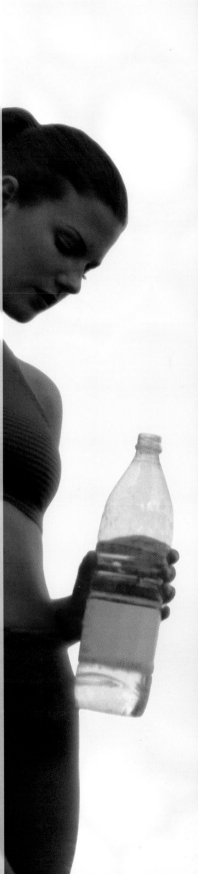

INTRODUCTION

Below: TATT-Doctor-speak for "tired all the time" – one of the major ailments in the 21st century.

How did you feel when you looked in the mirror this morning? Were you bright-eyed and bushy tailed, full of the joy of living and eager to begin a new day? Or did you reluctantly stumble into the bathroom, hoping that a shower would bring you back to life? You are not alone in feeling this way.

Despite the current pre-occupation with exercise and a healthy lifestyle, a lot of people are constantly tired, lethargic and depressed. In fact, one of the most common entries made on patients' records is TATT. That's doctor-speak for "tired all the time" – one of the major ailments in the 21st century. Like a lot of other people, you probably make frequent resolutions about exercise and diet, only to discover you are too tired to bother.

If you're a victim of TATT, there's probably a very simple reason for it. You are suffering from toxic overload, caused partly by the junk foods you consume and partly by the increasing number of pollutants that surround us all. Take heart. There is a cure.

YOU NEED A DETOX

Most people think of detoxing as a purely physical process, but there's more to it than dealing with bodily ills. If you're tired all the time, you obviously need to attend to your health. At the same time, it is now widely accepted that your physical well-being is inextricably interwoven with the state of your mind. This, of course, is affected by your surroundings, your home life and your employment.

In other words, a really thorough detox involves every aspect of your life. Yes, it is possible to detox your body without dealing with other aspects, but why settle for half measures? This book will explain how you can detox your body, your mind, your relationships and your surroundings.

Generally speaking, it's best to start with a body detox. Afterwards, you'll feel so much better that you'll be full of energy and enthusiasm to press on.

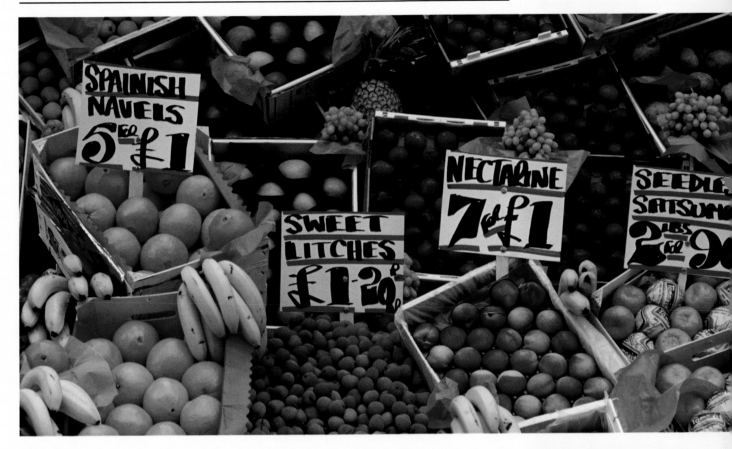

HOW LONG DOES IT TAKE?

The detoxification diets given in this book allow you to detox your body in 24 hours or in two days. Longer, more intensive programmes are available but, if you are new to detoxing, you are advised to begin with the safe and simple suggestions in the following pages.

A warning here – if you are pregnant, breast feeding, taking any type of medication, receiving any form of medical treatment or suffering from any illness, you should consult your GP before undertaking any of these recommendations.

THE PRACTICAL APPROACH

This book offers you the chance to change your life completely – and for the better. What's more, it's essentially practical. You don't need to buy expensive creams, lotions and equipment. The diets given don't include exotic ingredients. Everything you need can be obtained from your local supermarket – though you are advised to use organic produce if possible. The recipes given are easy to prepare and delicious to eat.

Above: everything you need can be obtained from your local supermarket – though you are advised to use organic produce if possible.

Take a look at the diet pages now, make out your shopping list and get started.

BUY A NOTEBOOK

You'll probably be so surprised and happy about the results of your physical detox that you'll be eager to go further with this project.

Before you begin the programmes for detoxing your mind and your relationships, you will need to buy an A4 hard-cover notebook with lined pages, and a supply of ballpoint pens. If you really do prefer to work on a computer, you can buy a supply of punched paper and a ring binder to hold it. Either choice can be used as your workbook. However, if you opt for the computer, remember to place a large green plant beside it on your desk.

Below: take a look at the diet pages now, make out your shopping list and get started.

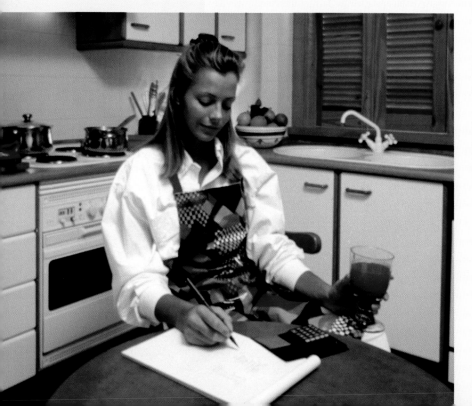

You'll probably find it easier and more pleasant to curl up on a comfortable sofa and to write by hand.

You may find a few startling suggestions in the MIND and RELATIONSHIPS sections. Don't dismiss them out of hand and say "I couldn't possibly …". You don't know what you can do until you try.

HOME SWEET HOME

You've probably heard of Feng Shui, so you won't be surprised that we recommend it in detoxing your home. If you find it difficult to accept that windchimes in your window can deflect bad chi (life energy), try it anyway. The delicate musical sounds are pleasant and if, by any chance, your fortunes should improve – well, it could be coincidence…

Why not place a money plant (*crassula argentea*) on your desk and see what happens?

Don't hesitate any longer. It's time to start on your big detoxification venture.

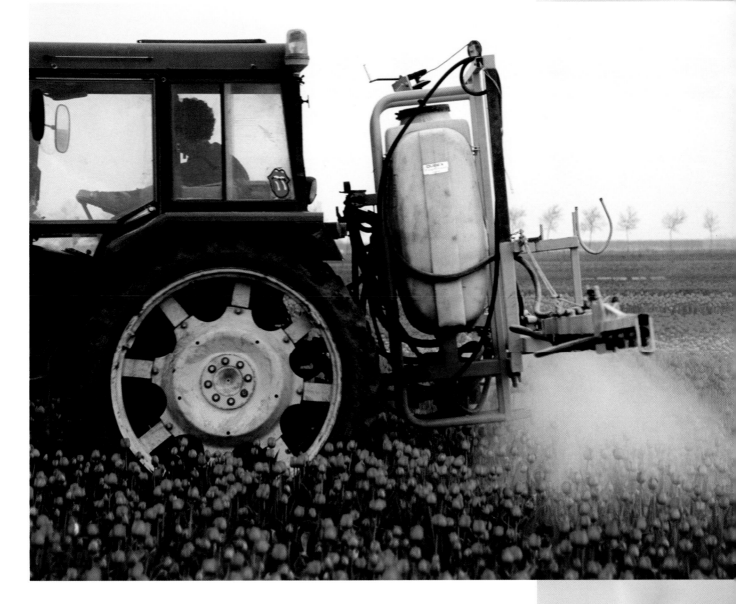

We need to detox our bodies because both inner and outer cleanliness are equally important to our well-being. In our fight against pollution and its associated ills, it's all too easy to forget this.

As we struggle to maintain immaculate surroundings we are actually increasing the toxins in our environment. We spray our homes with cleansers of various types, shake deodorising powders over our carpets, pour magic liquids into our toilet bowls – all of these contain chemicals that can cause a toxic reaction in our bodies. Remember, too, the various lotions and sprays with which we anoint ourselves. These also contain chemicals – and that equals more toxins.

Above: as we struggle to maintain immaculate surroundings we are actually increasing the toxins in our environment.

Below: toxins already in the atmosphere, created from exhaust fumes, factories, ventilation systems, industrial and agricultural chemicals, and tobacco smokers, to name but a few.

WHAT IS A TOXIN?

The medical definition of a toxin is "a poisonous protein produced by pathogenic bacteria". In the context of this book, a toxin is any substance that creates harmful or irritating effects in your body.

Unfortunately, toxins are not visible. If they were, perhaps we'd all be more vigilant about trying to avoid them.

Alarmingly, our 21st-century world is crammed with the things. Every time we use household cleansers or personal toiletries, we increase the toxins floating around – and then breathe them in. This is in addition to the toxins already in the atmosphere, created from exhaust fumes, factories, ventilation systems, industrial and agricultural chemicals, and tobacco smokers, to name but a few.

If you're reasonably healthy, your body will be able to handle a certain level of toxicity. Much depends, too, on your age. As we get older, our bodies have less resistance to the onslaught of toxins. Time passes, we become more vulnerable and health problems increase. Illnesses like arthritis, cancer, heart disease and tuberculosis are becoming more prevalent. More and more of us complain of vague aches and pains, colds, headaches, indigestion, stress, depression and the most common ailment of our time – constant tiredness.

Do toxins have anything to do with these conditions? According to the medical profession, the answer is "YES!" What's more, they are inescapable, even if you live in the heart of the country.

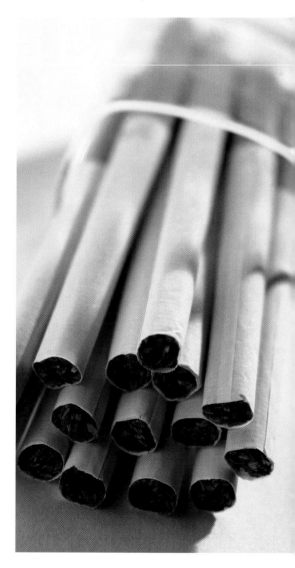

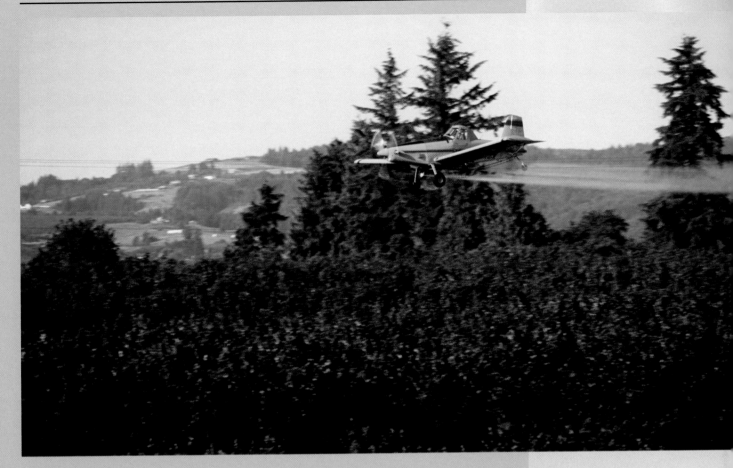

TOXINS ON YOUR PLATE

As we have already mentioned, the very air we breathe is laden with toxins. But that's not all. The meals we eat add to our daily intake. No matter how carefully we choose the food we buy, it's almost inevitable that it will contain chemicals in some shape or form. Farmers spray their crops, to protect them from pests and diseases. Systemic pesticides are applied to the earth where lettuces, carrots and other plants grow and infiltrate the flesh of the vegetables. What's more, washing or peeling has no effect. The residue of the pesticide remains actually inside the plant. Preservatives present another problem. These chemicals are widely used to protect the fruit or vegetable from deterioration in transit and during storage. Then there are the antibiotics and growth hormones used to make animals larger and to increase milk production. And what about the synthetic additives used to bleach, colour, preserve and flavour certain foods?

Above: farmers spray their crops, to protect them from pests and diseases.

NOT SO SAFE

We are assured, of course, that all this tampering with food is carefully monitored so that only a "safe level" of chemicals is present. That may be so. The fact remains that all the chemicals used add to the total toxicity in your body. And many chemicals once considered "safe" are now known to be harmful, even though some are still in everyday use.

Then, of course, there's genetic modification. Despite the welter of information to which we have been subjected, nobody seems to know very much about it. Or if they do, they're not telling. Like all the other weird and wonderful processes used on our food, most people regard it as highly suspect.

COOL, CLEAR WATER

Drinking about eight glasses of water every day is considered to be essential to health. And, surely, the consumption of so much liquid should flush any impurities from our bodie?. Alas – not necessarily.

Water, too, can be full of toxins. The production of tap water is strictly regulated, but there's always a risk of contamination from chemicals and heavy metals. Did you know that 50% of the nitrogen fertiliser used by farmers can seep into the water system?

Below: did you know that 50% of the nitrogen fertiliser used by farmers can seep into the water system?

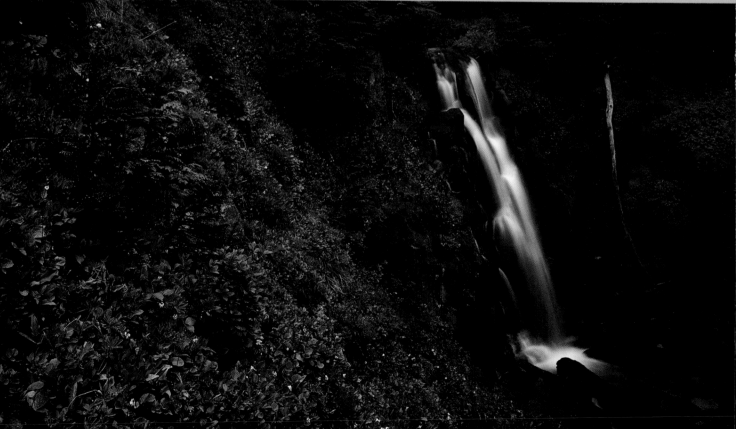

Furthermore, some of the "purifying" chemicals used by water companies are potentially damaging to your health. How many times have you turned on the tap and noticed a strong smell of chlorine? Some tap water smells – and tastes – like a swimming pool.

Incidentally, you can find out for yourself exactly what is used to process the drinking water in your area simply by contacting the water company and asking.

What about bottled spring water, fresh from the mountain streams? Well – perhaps. But we've all heard of the brands that turn out to be nothing more than carbonated tap water. And what about the filtering process to which bottled water is subjected?

Your best plan is probably to buy yourself a water filter. This can be as simple as a jug holding a cartridge which needs renewing every month, or as elaborate as a fitted system with a third tap above your sink.

Whichever method you choose, filtering is the best way to obtain drinking water of reasonable standard.

IN THE ENVIRONMENT

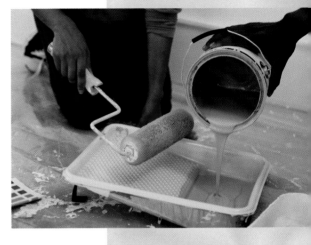

No matter how thoroughly you clean your home, it remains a source of toxins. They lurk not only in the chemical-laden cleansers you use, but in pollutants like dust, solvents and paints. If your home is not newly built, the paintwork could contain high levels of lead; there may even be asbestos linings to boiler cupboards and ducting.

SELF-PRODUCED TOXINS

On top of all the toxins we imbibe in one way or another, the body also produces toxins of its own, as break-down products of metabolism. These are the by-products called "free radicals" that can attack healthy cells and cause all sorts of problems.

Your own detoxification system can deal with these waste products but, over a period of time, they build up and can seriously affect your health. Remember that your body also deals with waste produced by internal bacteria, as well as the various parasites that live inside you.

Above: toxins lurk not only in the chemical-laden cleansers you use, but in pollutants like dust, solvents and paints.

STILL UNSURE?

Are you wondering if this is a lot of fuss about nothing? Sure – you get the occasional headache. When you're stressed, you feel tired and come out in spots. But these, surely, are common experienc?. A couple of painkillers or an early night will put matters right.

Below: most instances of feeling under the weather are linked with toxicity. Diet plays a leading roll in the toxic level of your body.

Most instances of feeling "under the weather" or constantly tired can be linked to toxicity. And yes – these are common experiences, but they don't need to be. Why not check out your toxicity levels? Each "yes" answer counts as one point.

Do you:

- *smoke?*
- *suffer from frequent headaches?*
- *get indigestion?*
- *have skin problems?*
- *feel tired all the time?*
- *have difficulty in concentrating?*
- *sleep badly?*
- *suffer from constipation?*
- *drink a lot of coffee or tea?*
- *eat white flour products?*
- *eat fried foods?*
- *sometimes indulge in too much alcohol?*
- *eat red meat?*
- *add salt to your meals?*
- *take sugar with cereals or drinks?*
- *live in a town or city?*
- *drive a car?*
- *use a mobile phone?*
- *work at a computer?*
- *live in a centrally heated, double glazed house?*
- *use household cleaning materials?*
- *live on a main road or near a power station?*
- *experience stress at work or at home?*
- *use make-up?*

Total

Now add up your marks. The higher your total score, the greater your level of toxicity.

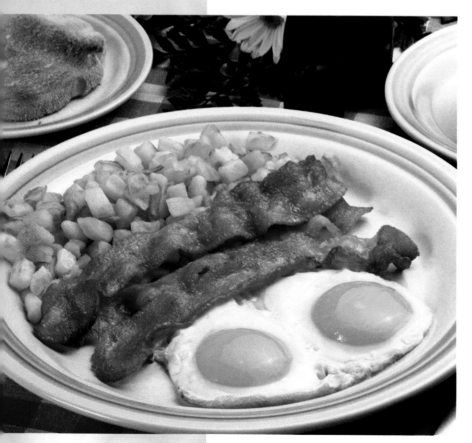

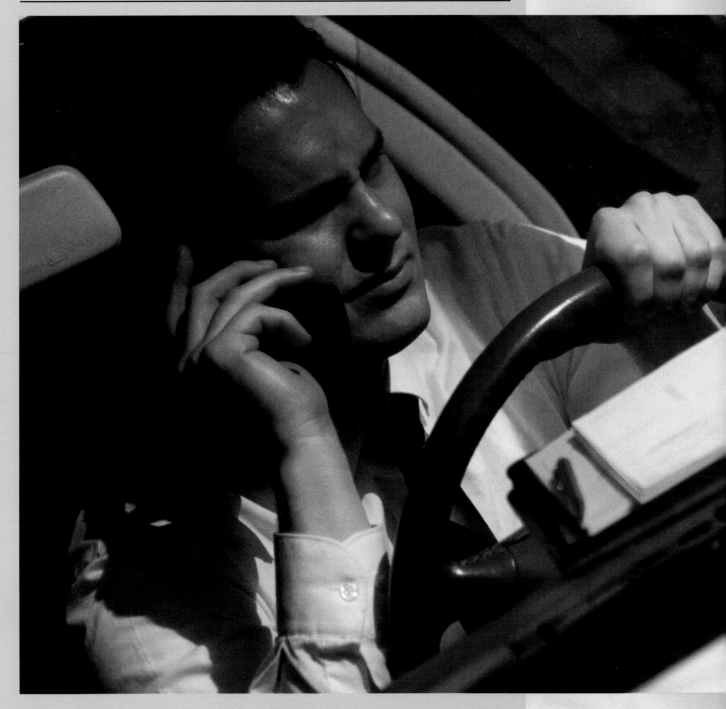

WHAT'S TO DO ABOUT IT?

Perhaps this all sounds very alarming. Having read this far, you may be thinking of escaping to a desert island. There's no need. It's easy to protect yourself from all the nasty things mentioned here. You simply need to invest in a detox.

Above: experience stress at work or at home?

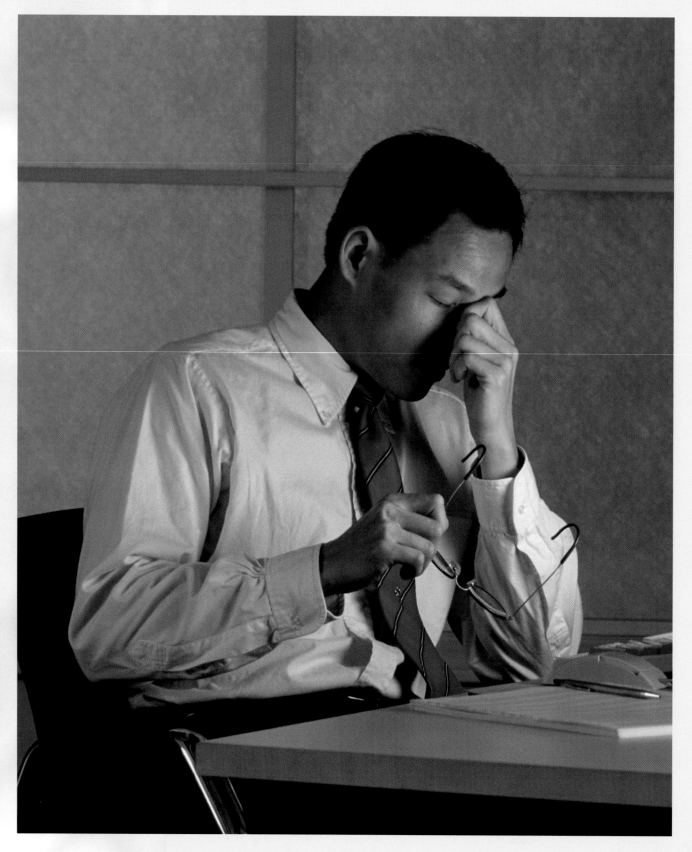

Your detoxification systems regularly go into battle, getting rid of all the toxins you have absorbed. There's no let-up in your body's fight against toxins. It goes on 24 hours every day.

THE RESPIRATORY AND IMMUNE SYSTEM

The respiratory system carries oxygen from the air to the bloodstream. It also expels waste products, such as carbon dioxide, that are formed as a result of the body's metabolism. The mucous membranes in your mouth and nose, plus the hairs in your nose and ears, are designed to protect your body from germs. White blood cells and antibodies attack any toxins or viruses that do get through these initial barricades.

The lungs have a dual role in the detox process. First, they remove toxins such as the carbon dioxide already mentioned. Second, they filter out the airborne pollutants that have escaped the initial filtering from the mucous membranes and hair in the nose.

THE GASTROINTESTINAL SYSTEM

Every morsel of food you eat passes through your stomach to the intestines. Here the nutrients are absorbed and waste matter is abandoned for elimination. This is the bowels' role – a healthy bowel shifts large quantities of waste every day.

The liver, too, is engaged in the detoxification exercise. It deals with bacteria, yeasts, viruses, parasites and a wide variety of other invaders. Once neutralised, these waste products are transferred to the intestines and from there to the bowels, where they are excreted.

Far left: there's no let-up in your body's fight against toxins. It goes on 24 hours every day.

Below: your detoxification systems regularly go into battle, getting rid of all the toxins you have absorbed.

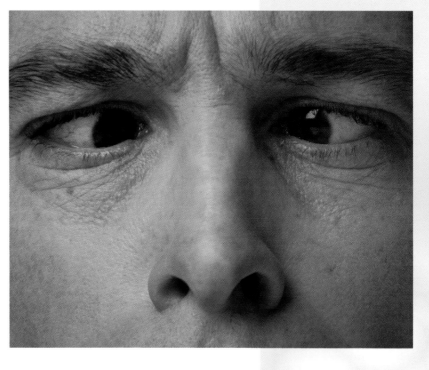

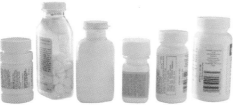

Right: all the systems of the body have a roll to play in filtering the toxins absorbed during day-to-day life.

THE URINARY SYSTEM

The kidneys, too, have an important job to do by filtering out toxins in the blood and eliminating them through urine. They also recycle valuable nutrients for future use by the body.

THE LYMPHATIC SYSTEM

Your body's waste disposal system has another ally in the elaborate network of vessels comprising the lymphatic system. It runs alongside the bloodstream, delivering nutrients to every cell in the body and eliminating waste. Lymph nodes are found behind your knees, under your arms, in your groin, stomach and throat. As the lymph vessels pass through these nodes, waste matter is filtered out.

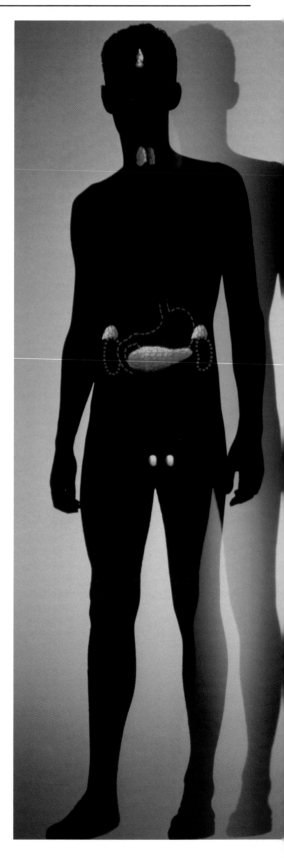

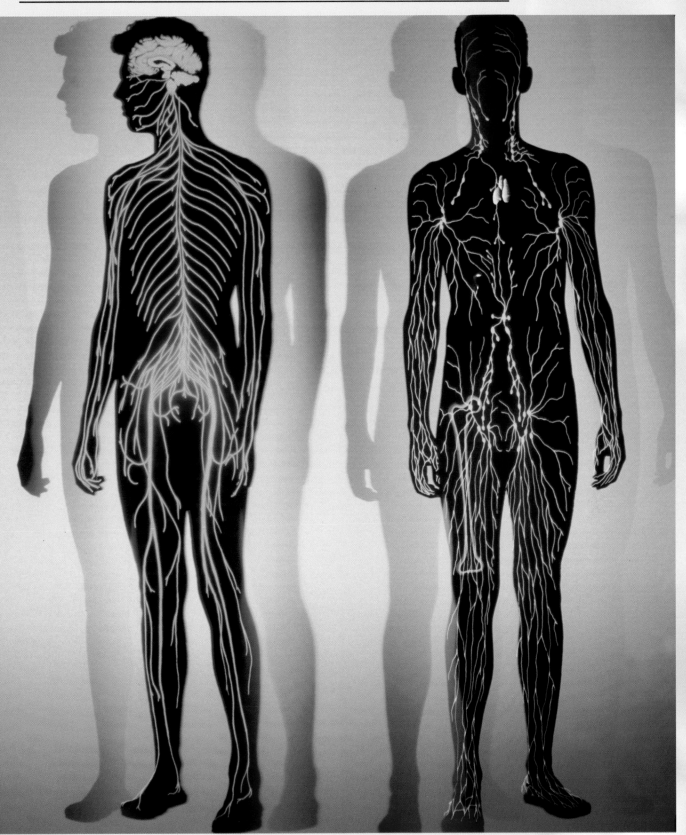

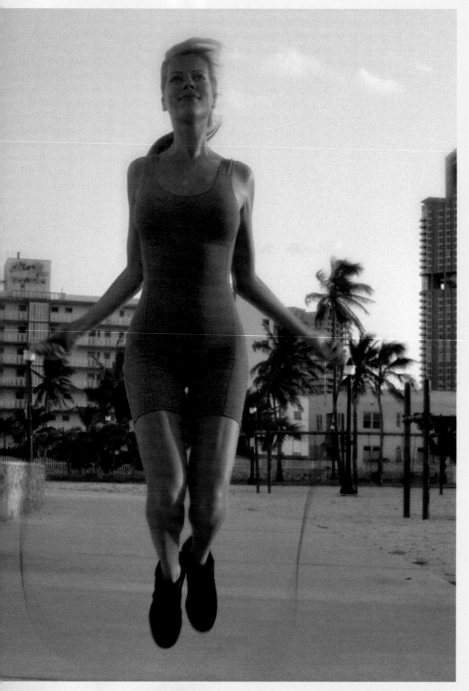

Above: when you sweat, for instance, your skin is allowing toxins to be expelled.

THE SKIN

Your skin is the largest organ in your body and it's essential to detoxification. When you sweat, for instance, your skin is allowing toxins to be expelled.

Detoxification systems

Respiratory and immune
Throat, sinuses, immune nose and lungs

Gastrointestinal
Liver, colon, gastrointestinal tract

Urinary
Kidneys, bladder, urethra

Lymphatic
Lymph vessels and nodes

Skin
Sebaceous glands

Do you need to detox?

Are you wondering why, if your body makes such a splendid job of the detoxification process, there is any need for you to take an active part?

As was said earlier, we can all cope with a certain level of toxicity. However, there are times – particularly when you have been under stress or feel tired – when you absorb far more toxins than your body can cope with. It needs some help from you. Even a one-day detox can make a dramatic improvement in the way you feel. So make up your mind to undertake this simple project as soon as possible.

When is the best time to detox?

It is generally agreed that the best times to detox are in the spring or the autumn, but this is not always possible. Realistically, you should undertake this venture when you have a few days to spare. Choose a time when you can stay at home, perhaps a weekend or when you have a holiday. A detox, even if only of one day's duration, is a full time occupation. Undertaking your first detox and working at the same time is not advisable.

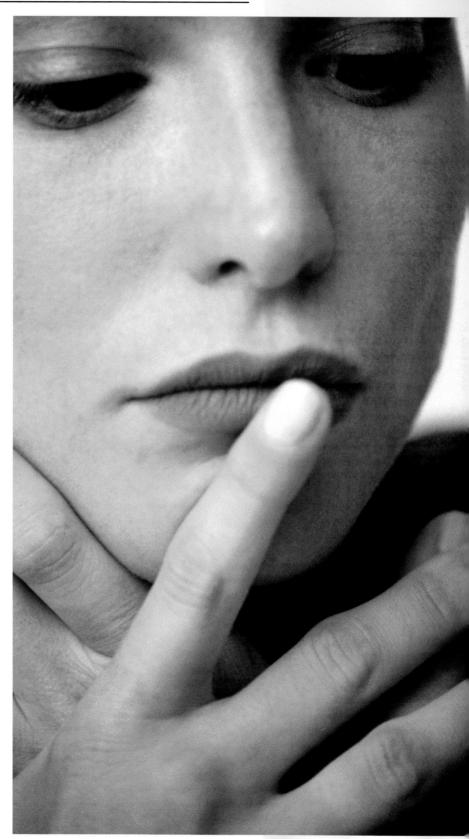

Below: have a shopping trip the day before you begin your detox and stock up with the things you need.

SO HOW DO I GO ABOUT IT?

First, as stated above, be sure that you have two or three days off work. Choose a time, too, when you are feeling in an upbeat frame of mind and are not under stress. Try to select a date two or three weeks ahead, so that you will be able to make the necessary preparations.

Having selected a date for your detox, begin to change the way you eat and drink. Try not to smoke at all. If you must, cut down drastically on the number of cigarettes you smoke every day. Similar comments apply to alcohol, coffee, tea and other stimulants. Reduce your intake of fats and sugar. Eat more fresh fruit, vegetables and salads. Drink as much water and fruit juice as you can.

Next – go through your kitchen cupboards and throw out all processed, fatty, sugary, or salty foods.

The fourth preparatory step is to make a collection of magazines, books and videos to occupy your time. During the detox period, you need to reward yourself for being strong-minded.

Fifth – consult an holistic practitioner or your GP before undertaking the detox. Ask their advice about taking a lactobacillus acidophilus supplement throughout your detox period, to guard against constipation and diarrhoea.

Sixth – have a shopping trip the day before you begin your detox and stock up with the things you need.

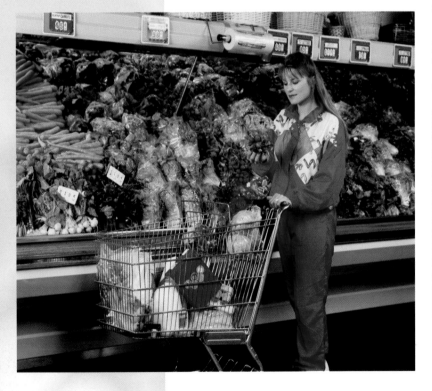

Shopping list

Vegetables
Broccoli, cabbage, carrots, celery, lettuce, onions

Fruits
Grapes, apples, kiwi, mango, peaches, pears

Drinks
Herbal teas, still mineral water

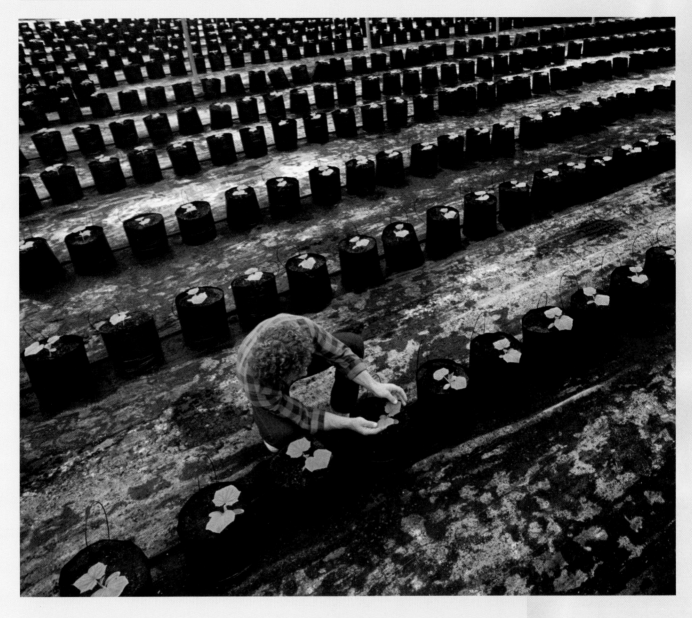

FOODS TO AVOID

The aim of a detox is to alkalise the system, so steer clear of oranges, lemons, grapefruit and pineapples. Don't eat dried fruit; it contains the chemical called sulphur dioxide. It's best, too, not to eat bananas. They contain a lot of starch and are mucous forming.

GO ORGANIC

If at all possible, buy organic fruit and vegetables. These are free from chemical fertilisers and insecticides. Most supermarkets now stock organic products, but if you can find a local supplier this will be even better.

Above: if at all possible, buy organic fruit and vegetables.

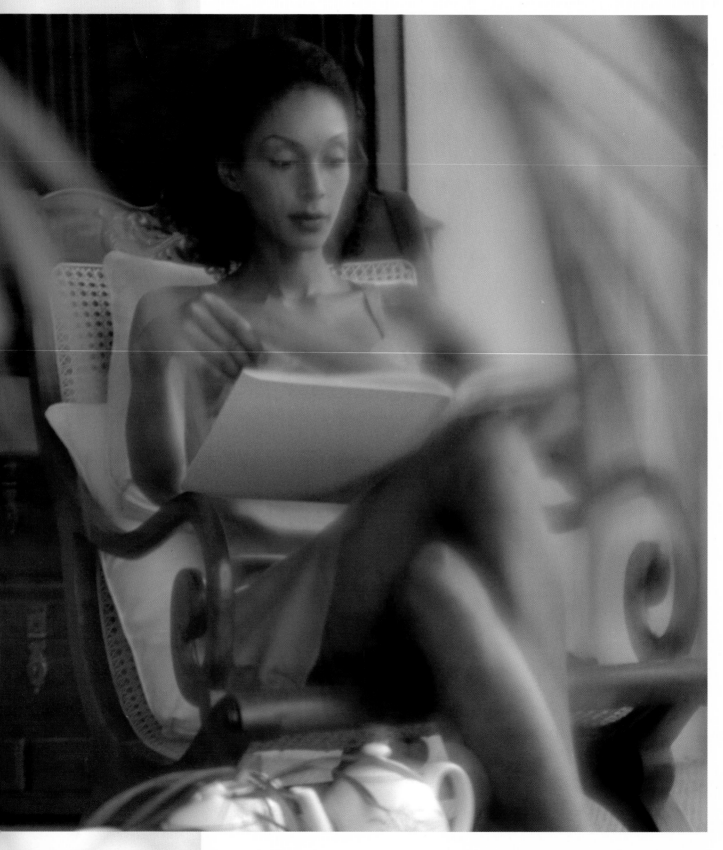

Y ou've done your shopping, stocked up with reading matter, videos and CDs. It's time for the off. First, though, one point must be made clear:

A detox is not the same as a fast

During a fast, nothing except water passes your lips. All other food and drink is banned. A detox programme is less drastic. You are allowed to eat and drink throughout the procedure, but you must stick with the prescribed menus. Do not, on any account, be tempted to cut down on the meals suggested or miss them out entirely. You'll simply make yourself feel wretched.

And, by the way, a detox is not a weight-loss programme, either. You will almost certainly lose a few pounds in the process, but the weight lost will swiftly return once you get back to normal eating patterns.

Far left: you are allowed to eat and drink throughout the procedure, but you must stick with the prescribed menus.

Below: it's time for the off.

Below: on waking drink a cup of herbal tea or a glass of hot water.

ONE-DAY DIETS

There are two types of one-day diets. The first is the **One-Day Cleansing Diet.** This gentle introduction to detox is recommended for your first attempt. Not only does it cleanse the system and give your digestion a rest, it's especially helpful if you normally eat red meat, smoke or drink.

On waking
A cup of herbal tea or a glass of hot water.

Breakfast
As much raw fruit as you wish to satisfy your appetite. Restrict the fruit to the list given earlier and be sure to chew it well.

Elevenses
A cup of herbal tea or fresh fruit juice.

Lunch
Make up a vegetable salad. Choose from lettuce, red/white cabbage, broccoli, grated carrots, cauliflower florets, chopped onions, chicory, endive, cress and beetroot. Sprinkle with herbs. Chew well and eat slowly.

Dinner
A vegetable salad, as above. For dessert, select one of the permitted fruits. Or you can chop up two or three and make into a fruit salad.

Bedtime
A cup of herbal tea, such as camomile or peppermint, will help to soothe you to sleep.

NB: Throughout the day, drink as much plain clear water as you wish.

DON'T PICK

However hungry you may feel, it is not a good idea to "pick" at various foods, even those listed, between meals. The whole idea of this programme is to give your digestive system and liver a rest. Snacking – even if only on a few grapes or half an apple – defeats the object.

THE ONE-DAY MONO DIET

On a mono diet, you eat only one type of food throughout the day. You can choose from raw fruit, raw vegetables or cooked food, but you must not mix them. This diet permits mini-meals throughout the day, eaten at intervals of about two hours.

Raw fruit allowed
Apples, grapes, pears, papaya.

Raw vegetables allowed
Carrots, cabbage, celery, cucumber.

Cooked food allowed
Brown rice, buckwheat, millet, potatoes.

Drink throughout the day
Plain water or herbal teas. To avoid dehydration, ensure that you drink a minimum of two litres of still mineral water or filtered water. Don't down a glass at one go. Sip the water. That way, you won't notice how much more than usual you are drinking.

Breakfast
If you're following the raw fruit or raw vegetable diet, be sure to wash each item carefully.

For the cooked food diet, boil the cereal or potatoes in unsalted water. Make a dressing with a teaspoonful of olive and oil and squeeze of lemon juice.

11am Your mid-morning meal, as above. Remember that you must not mix the diets. Stick with raw fruit or raw vegetables or cooked food.

1pm Another mini-meal for lunch. Ring the changes by chopping the fruit or vegetables. If you're on the cooked food diet, try mashing the potatoes and sprinkling with herbs.

4pm Tea time. Have another mini-meal.

6pm Mini-meal supper.

Bedtime drink
Herbal tea or hot water. Be sure to have a glass of water beside your bed, in case you feel thirsty during the night.

Below: the mono diet allows you only one type of food throughout the day – raw or cooked, but not a mixture.

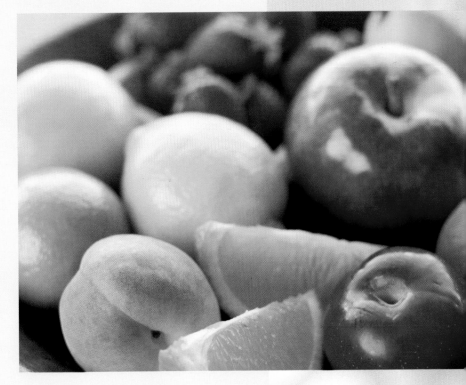

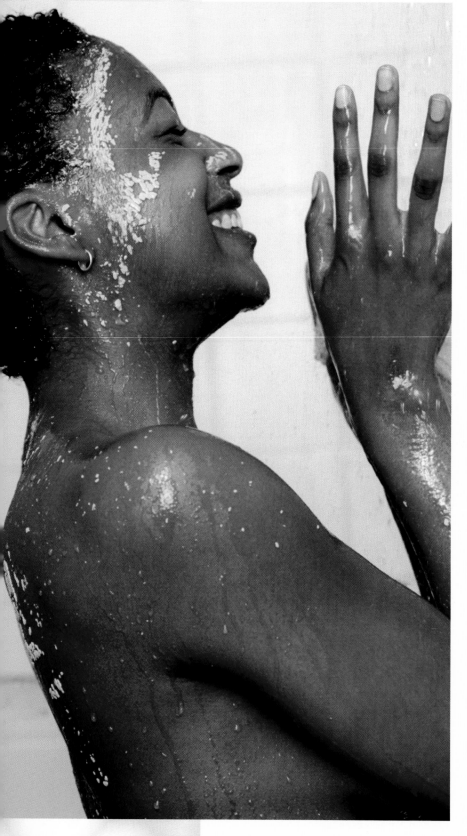

The morning after

When you wake up next morning, you have every right to feel pleased with yourself. And it won't take long for you to realise that you really do feel different – relaxed, clean and revitalised. Savour that feeling for a few minutes before you get out of bed.

Then stand at an open window, have a good long stretch and take some deep breaths of fresh air. A shower comes next – or why not indulge yourself with a warm, luxuriously scented bath?

Having been on a diet for 24 hours, you probably won't fancy a full, fried breakfast. Even if you do – resist the temptation. Instead, choose some fruit and natural yogurt, and a glass of fruit juice. If you feel hungry, you may have a slice of wholemeal toast.

For the next couple of days eat sparingly and steer clear of coffee, tea, alcohol and soft drinks. Don't be surprised if you lose interest in heavy meals, gooey desserts, chocolate and all the other "sinful" things you used to enjoy. Instead, you'll develop an addiction to the wonderfully clear, clean feeling that results from even a one-day detox. You may even decide that, next time you have time off from work, you will treat yourself to a longer detox.

HOW ABOUT A TWO-DAY DETOX?

This one is especially beneficial if you're exhausted after a period of stress and tension.

Getting ready

As before, aim to start your detox a couple of weeks ahead. That way you'll have time to prepare for it. For a week before you start, reduce your intake of red meat, coffee, tea and alcohol. If you didn't stop smoking after the One-Day Cleansing Diet, now is the time to kick the habit.

TWO-DAY DETOX

FIRST DAY

When you wake, pour a glass of hot water, add the juice of half a lemon and sip it slowly.

For the rest of the day, eat black or white grapes whenever you wish. Ideally, eat a kilo, throughout the day.

Drink fresh fruit or vegetable juices, herbals teas and – of course – LOTS of still mineral water or filtered tap water. Dilute fruit juices with water.

SECOND DAY

When you wake, drink a glass of hot water with the juice of half a lemon.

For the rest of the day, you should eat apples – as many as you like, but aim for a minimum of eight.

Drink – as always – plenty of water, herbal teas, vegetable juices and diluted fruit juices.

Far left: even after just one day of detox you will feel relaxed, clean and revitalised.

Below: eat black or white grapes whenever you wish. Ideally, eat a kilo, throughout the day.

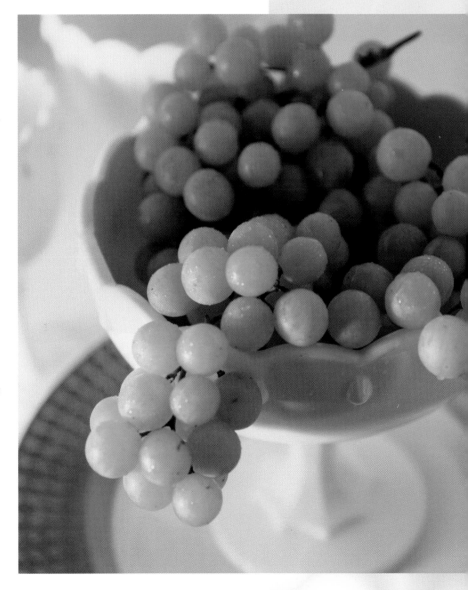

Below: for insomnia releif, try soaking in a warm, lavender-scented bath for half an hour, then go to bed.

Fer right: soon after your detox you'll be more alert and energetic.

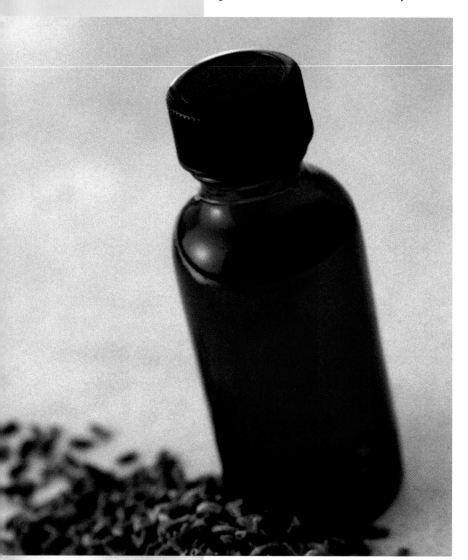

LONGER DIETS

A number of longer, more intensive detox diets exist and these can be very beneficial. However, if you intend to undertake a detox programme lasting more than three days, you will be well advised to do this under the supervision of a qualified nutritionist, naturopath or your GP. Any of these practitioners will probably be willing to prescribe a suitable diet for you.

WHAT ABOUT SIDE-EFFECTS?

You are unlikely to suffer from side-effects with a one- or two-day detox. The longer programmes are a different matter. The detoxification process releases into your system the overload of toxins it has been unable to deal with. This means – sorry! – that you may feel pretty sick at times. So what can you expect?

Headaches
Don't be tempted to use painkillers. Instead, drink a spoonful of honey dissolved in hot water. Close your eyes and relax as much as possible.

Constipation
Drink lots of water, but not with meals. Eat slowly and chew your food thoroughly.

Diarrhoea
Drink even more water. If the condition lasts for more than 36 hours, consult your doctor.

Insomnia
Soak in a warm, lavender-scented bath for half an hour, then go to bed.
Put two drops of lavender oil on a tissue and place it under your pillow.
Drink a cup of camomile tea before you put out the light, then snuggle down and listen to a relaxation tape.

Nausea
Drink a cup of ginger tea.

Body odour and bad breath
Brush your teeth and tongue
regularly. Gargle with a gentle
mouthwash.

Shivering, feeling cold
Turn up the heating and wrap
yourself in a blanket. A hot drink
will warm you.

IT'S WORKING!

However wretched you may feel,
these and other minor problems,
such as depression and mood
swings, are signs that the detox is
working well. All the woes you are
suffering indicate that the toxins
are being thrown out of your
system. Resolve that, once this
programme is over, you will never
again allow yourself to reach such a
high level of toxicity.

WORTH THE EFFORT

Soon after your detox, you will
notice some marked differences in
the way you feel. You'll be more
alert and energetic. The condition
of your skin and hair will improve
markedly. Almost certainly, you
will decide that – despite the minor
problems – the effort was
worthwhile.

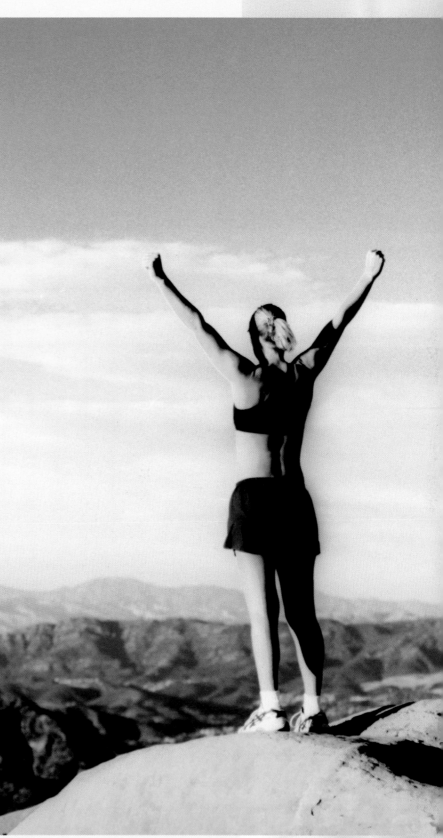

BREATHING

One way in which chemicals attack your body is via the lungs. As you breathe, you inhale hundreds of toxic molecules and particles that enter your bloodstream almost immediately. It's a sobering thought, isn't it, that as you breathe you inhale at least a fraction of everything around you. Exhaust fumes, industrial waste, smoke, other people's germs – all these and many other pollutants assail your body with every breath you take.

WHAT TO DO ABOUT IT

Oxygen – which exists even in the polluted air of inner cities – is vital to life. You can live for several days without food and water. Without oxygen, you die within minutes. On no account should you stop breathing.It's seldom necessary to wear a mask, either.

Don't worry. There are ways of counteracting the problems of pollution. For example, you can certainly improve the quality of the air you breathe in your own home. To begin with, invest in an ioniser.

This little machine changes the electrical charge of the atmosphere in a room so that its quality matches seaside air. If some of your colleagues are smokers, maybe you should set up an ioniser at work, too. You can try asking them not to smoke, but this may make you decidedly unpopular.

However, you can make your own home a No Smoking zone. Get into the habit, too, of opening doors and windows wide, at least two or three times a day, even in cold weather.

Below: oxygen – which exists even in the polluted air of inner cities – is vital to life.

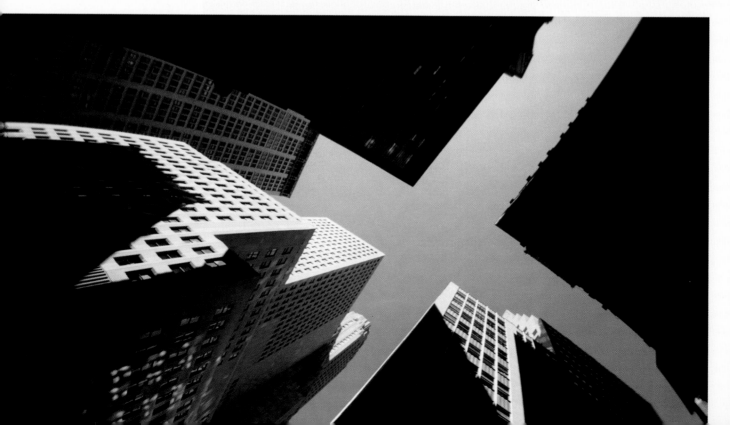

AN APPLE A DAY

Recent research indicates that eating just one apple a day enhances the health of your lungs. Apples contain an antioxidant called quercitin that enhances the respiratory system. Similar beneficial effects are also found in onions, tea and red wine.

Other fruits – cherries, blueberries, raspberries, blackberries and other dark red berries – also benefit your breathing.

HOW DO YOU BREATHE?

Generally speaking, the only people who regularly give any thought to their breathing are sufferers from asthma, emphysema and other respiratory problems. Most of us don't even notice the habitual regular cycles of inhale/exhale. We notice our breathing only when the lift is out of order and we need to climb several flights of stairs or when we have to run to catch a bus. Panting, we gasp, "I should take more exercise." But we don't actually do anything about it.

Spend a few minutes right now paying attention to the way you breathe. Is your breathing quick and shallow? Health experts say that most people's shallow breathing fills only the top quarter of their lungs. If this is how you

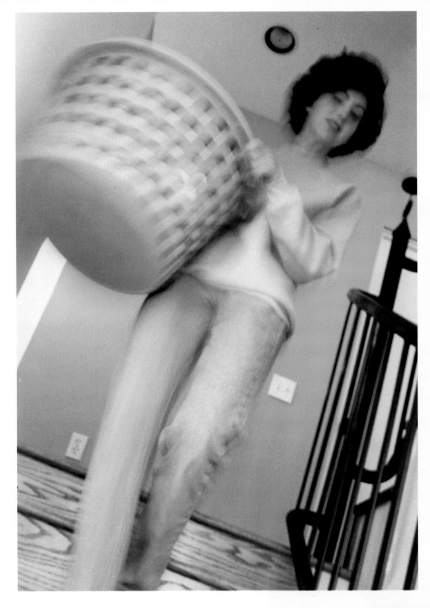

breathe, you're probably expelling only half the waste products you inhale.

This means that whenever you take a new breath, old air remains in your lungs and is pushed deeper into the body. In consequence, the level of oxygen circulating in your body is significantly reduced.

Above: most of us only notice our breathing when the lift is out of order and we need to climb several flights of stairs or when we have to run to catch a bus.

breathe, you're probably expelling only half the waste products you inhale.

This means that whenever you take a new breath, old air remains in your lungs and is pushed deeper into the body. In consequence, the level of oxygen circulating in your body is significantly reduced.

DIAPHRAGM OR CHEST?

What happens when you breathe? Do you lift your chest and your rib cage? Or do you breathe from your diaphragm? It's easy to find out.

1 Lie on your back on the floor.

2 Place one hand flat on your chest and the other on your stomach.

3 Continue to breathe normally, but keep your attention on your hands. Which one moves first?

If the hand on your chest moves first, you are not using your lungs as you should.

Below: lying flat on your back, keep the rhythm flowing and you will swiftly drift into sleep.

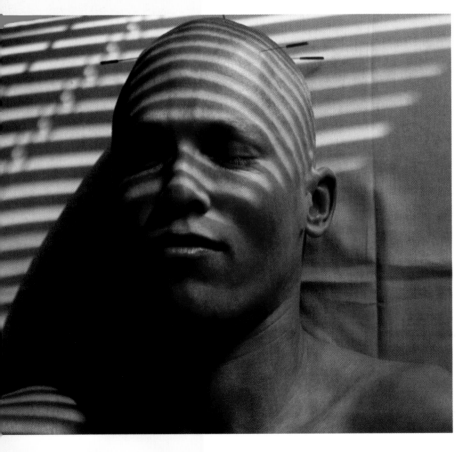

YOGA BREATHING EXERCISES

Correct breathing is of primary importance in the practice of some therapies, particularly those originating in the East. In yoga, the air is believed to contain prana, the life force. Correct breathing increases your intake of this vital energy.

For this reason, yoga includes a number of breathing exercises. You may care to try the two below.

EXERCISE 1– FULL BREATHING

1 Lie flat on your back – either on the floor or on your bed. If you have back problems, push a rolled up towel under your lower back or place a small cushion beneath your knees.

2 Rest your hands on your abdomen, just above your navel.

3 Close your eyes.

4 When you are ready, inhale deeply and slowly into your diaphragm, allowing your hands to be gently lifted.

5 Exhale slowly, lightly pressing your abdomen.

6 Repeat this exercise five times, gradually increasing to 15 repetitions.

NB: When you finish the repetitions, remain still for a few minutes. If you jump up quickly, you may feel dizzy. During the exercise, take particular notice of the rhythm of the abdomen rising as you inhale and contracting as you exhale.

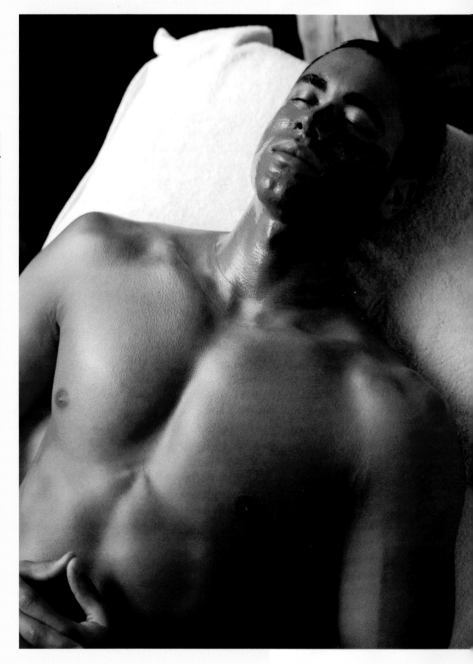

Below: Full Breathing can be practised best when you have a little time to relax and lie down either on your bed or on the floor.

EXERCISE 2 –
ALTERNATE NOSTRIL BREATHING

This exercise is particularly useful for clearing stale air and waste products from the lungs and body. It increases your energy, balances your mind and strengthens the respiratory system.

Sit upright on a straight-backed chair or cross-legged on the floor.

1 Close your right nostril with your right thumb. Exhale through your left nostril.

2 Inhale through your left nostril to a count of four.

3 Close your left nostril with the ring and little finger of your right hand. The index and middle fingers should rest on the bridge of your nose. Inhale through your right nostril. Hold to a count of 16.

4 Release the right nostril and exhale to a count of eight.

5 Keep your left nostril closed and inhale through your right nostril to a count of four.

6 Keep both nostrils closed for a count of 16.

7 Release your left nostril. Exhale to a count of eight.

8 Start again with step 2 above. Repeat the whole sequence 10 times. Breathe in to a count of four, hold the breath for a count of 16 and exhale to a count of eight.

NB: When you first try this exercise, you may feel dizzy. If this happens, take a break and continue when you feel able. Stop at once if you find it difficult to maintain an even rhythm.

Below: alternate nostril breathing is particularly good at clearing stale air from the lungs.

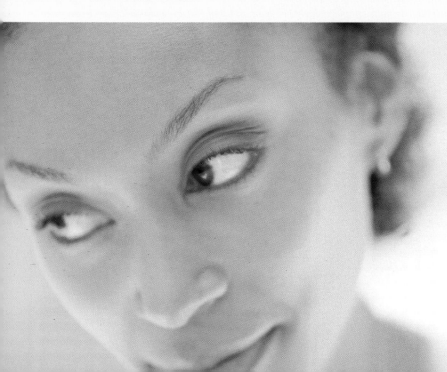

If you practise these exercises every day, you will soon find that your breathing becomes slower and deeper. This will enhance the function and capacity of your lungs and assist with the expulsion of toxins. Practitioners of yoga also believe that the exercises increase the flow of prana (life energy) throughout your body.

EXERCISE

Most experts agree that we need at least 30 minutes of physical exercise, five times a week. This is a great way to relieve stress and to increase the flow of oxygen to the brain. It stimulates our bodies to shed toxins, as well as toning our muscles, strengthening our bones and guarding against heart disease.

Aerobic exercise is particularly beneficial and it's easy to fit into your daily life. Use the stairs instead of the lift; walk briskly instead of taking the car and put more effort into everything you do, whether it's pushing a vacuum cleaner over the carpet or a mower over the lawn.

If you're not into the gym scene, choose two or three activities that you enjoy – cycling, swimming, running, dancing – and practise them regularly. These will work different muscle groups and the variety will keep you interested.

One of the popular bodywork therapies, like yoga, tai chi, shiatsu or pilates may appeal to you. All of these can be practised at home, but it's best to attend classes to start with, to ensure that you learn the correct movements.

Regular exercise is an important detoxing tool. Try to incorporate it into your everyday life. However, it's not a good idea to start a new exercise routine while you are actually undertaking a detox.

Try to take a brisk daily walk and, if you wish, this can be supplemented by stretching. This is often overlooked as a form of exercise, but it can refresh and relax you at any time, and is a great stress-buster.

Below: regular exercise is an important detoxing tool. Try to incorporate it into your everyday life.

STRETCHING OUT

The great advantage of stretching as an exercise is that you don't need any special equipment and it can be done anywhere at any time.

Start the day with stretching – you don't even have to get out of bed to do it. Throw back the duvet and begin. Gentle stretching first thing in the morning gets the blood pumping through your body and wakes up your brain cells for the day ahead.

Stretch during the day, too. Take a quick stretch whenever you leave your desk or have a break of any kind, however brief. Stretch up to that high shelf, instead of getting a stool to stand on. Reach out to pass a file to a colleague, instead of leaving your desk to take it to him. You will be surprised how easy it is to fit stretching into your life.

FITNESS STRETCHES

The following four stretches will improve your stamina and your balance, increase your lung capacity and boost your energy levels.

1. MOUNTAIN POSTURE
Stand upright, your weight distributed evenly, with legs straight. Lift the pelvic floor, roll the collar bone up. Stretch the arms, hands and fingers up and to the sides, keeping them parallel to the ground. Keeping the head balanced and straight, roll the shoulders back. As you stretch the arms, widen the chest and breathe deeply. Take 10 slow deep breaths.

1

2. KNEE LIFT

Standing upright, bend the left knee up. Pull the heel close to the left buttock, keeping the right leg and foot strong, the right arm relaxed. Keep collar bones level, relax the neck and hold the head straight. Breathe deeply and hold the posture for 60 seconds. Release, relax and repeat the moves on the other side.

3. QUAD STRETCH

Standing upright, pull your left foot behind the back and towards the buttock. Keep lifting the pelvic floor and ensure the collar bones are at equal height. Focus your eyes on a point ahead, to maintain your balance. Breathe deeply, holding the posture for 60 seconds. Relax, then repeat the moves on the other side.

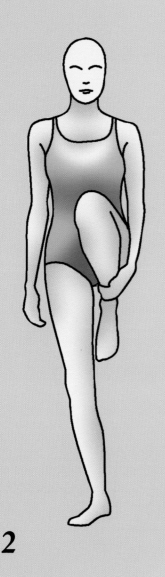

2

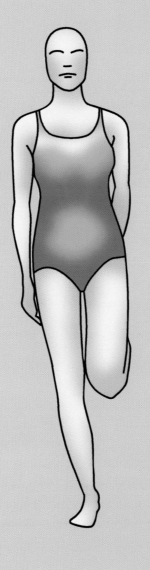

3

Right: be aware of your breath as you do each exercise.

4. QUAD AND BODY STRETCH
Hold your left foot behind your back, pulling the foot up and towards the buttock. Keep the right leg straight and stretch the right arm straight up. Remain balanced and centred, breathing deeply, for 60 seconds. Repeat on the other side.

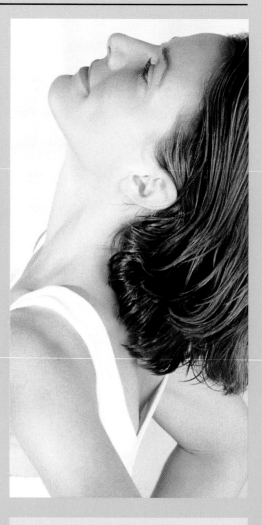

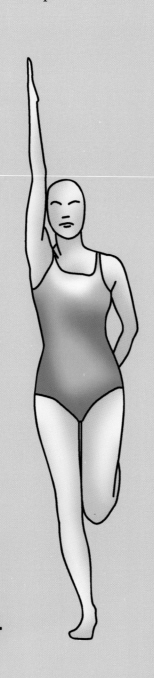

4

CORRECT BREATHING

- *Be aware of your breath as you do each exercise.*

- *Breathe slowly and evenly.*

- *Exhale as your stretch out, inhale as you retract.*

- *Consciously relax your muscles as you breathe.*

- *Breathe into the diaphragm, not the upper chest.*

SALUTE TO THE SUN

This popular yoga exercise increases your flexibility, boosts the oxygen in your bloodstream, stimulates your digestion and encourages the elimination of toxins. At first, you may find it difficult to learn this routine but it is well worth persevering. Once learned, the Salute to the Sun postures produce an almost balletic sequence.

1. *Stand with feet hip-width apart, arms hanging by your sides. Imagine that a piece of string attached to your crown is pulling your head towards the ceiling.*

2. *As you inhale, raise your arms out to the sides, bringing your palms together directly above your head. At the end of the in-breath, look up at your hands.*

3. *Exhale and, folding from the hips, bend down to touch the floor. (If you can't manage this, touch your thighs,)*

4. *Inhale, bending your knees so that you can place both palms flat on the floor on either side of your feet.*

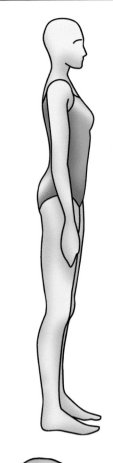

1

2

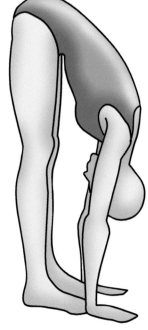

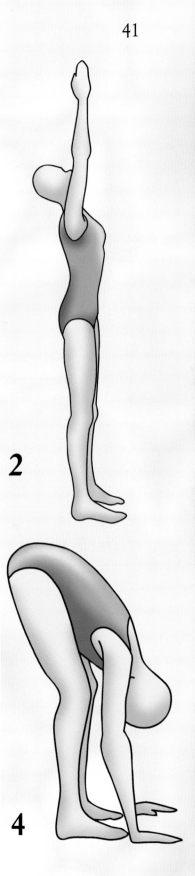

3

4

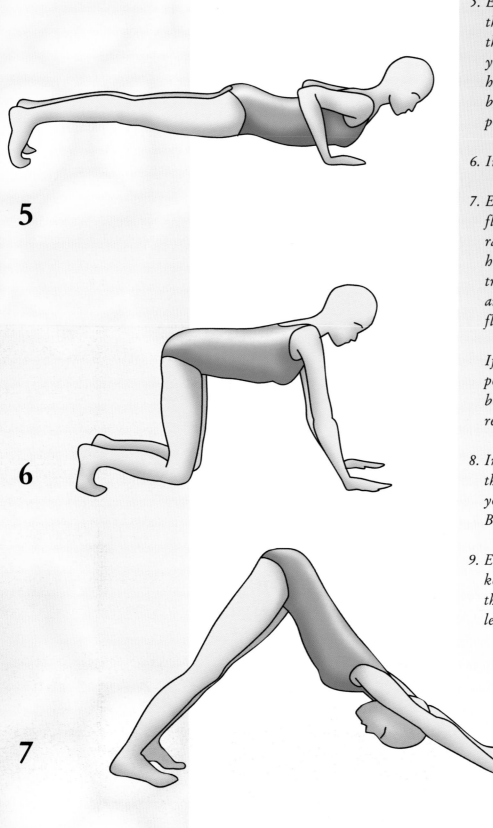

5

6

7

5. *Exhale. Step both feet back so that you are lying face down on the floor, legs extended with your toes tucked under. Your hands should be flat on the floor beside your ribcage, elbows pointing upwards.*

6. *Inhale and come up on all fours.*

7. *Exhale. Push away from the floor. Straighten your legs and raise your hips, keeping your head down so that you make a triangle with the floor. Your feet and heels should be flat on the floor.*

If you wish, you may hold this position for three to five breaths before repeating the sequence in reverse.

8. *Inhale. Step your feet forward so that they are again between your hands (as in position 4). Bend your knees if necessary.*

9. *Exhale and straighten your legs, keeping your fingers touching the floor or the backs of your legs (as in position 3).*

10. Inhale, then straighten up, raising your arms in a circle and placing your palms together directly over your head (as in position 2). At the end of the in-breath, look up towards your hands.

11. Exhale, dropping your hands to the sides. Look straight ahead (as in position 1).

SYNCHRONISATION

Once you have mastered this routine, it may be repeated as often as you wish. Salute to the Sun can be used as a warm-up or as an aerobic exercise. It all depends on how quickly you perform it. Remember that, whatever speed you take it, the movements should be synchronised with your breathing.

NB: There are many versions of Salute to the Sun. This is a short one, but if you prefer to perform the full traditional routine details can be found in almost any book about yoga.

TAKING A WALK

You have already been advised to take a walk every day. The exercise, and being in the fresh air, will be beneficial. Ideally, you should warm up at the start of your walk by strolling at a fairly slow pace. When you feel ready, increase the pace for as long as you wish, but remember to slow down again in order to cool off before your walk finishes.

POINTS TO REMEMBER

Maintain a good posture.

Keep your head up, and your shoulders in line with your hips.

Swing your arms in a natural rhythm.

If you like to walk to music, sing softly to yourself rather than using a mobile radio. You don't want to miss the rustle of the leaves, the song of the birds or the sigh of the surf on the shore.

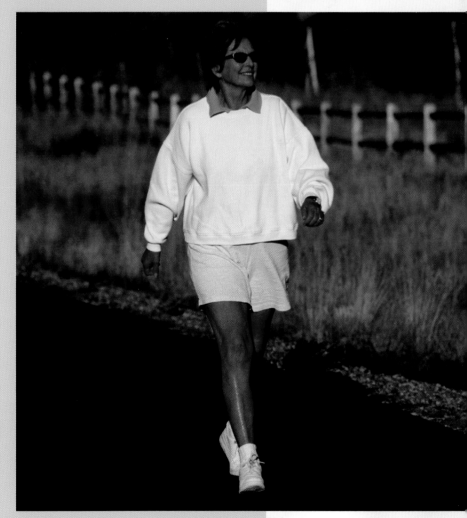

Below: take a walk every day.

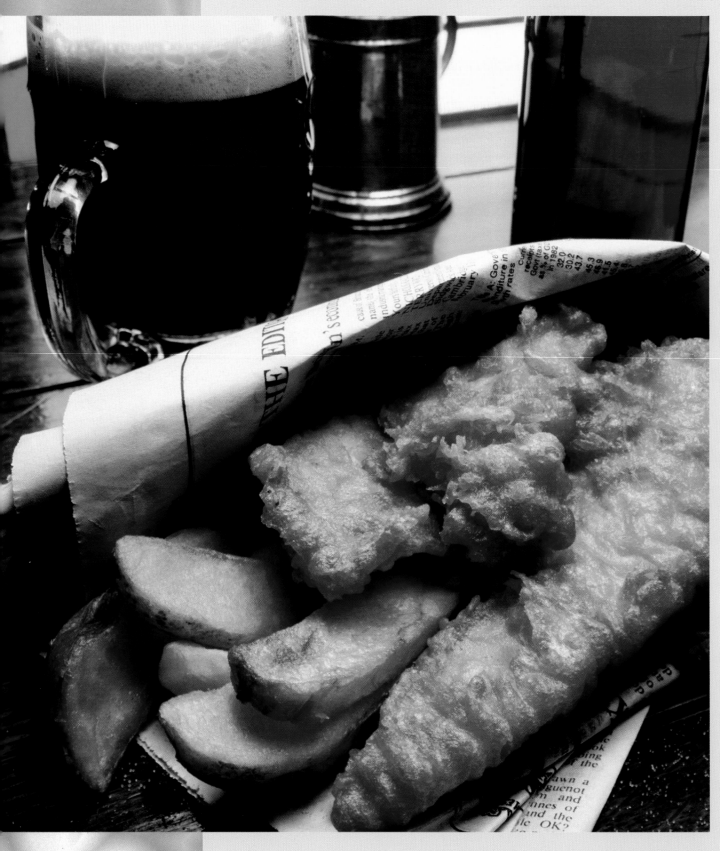

Health and vitality come from the food we eat, yet a lot of people consider themselves well fed if they always have "three good meals a day". This usually translates as a breakfast fry-up, and, at lunch time, a meal at the pub – probably meat pie and chips.

On the way home from work, they'll collect a take-away Chinese or Indian meal. Fluid intake for the day is likely to include strong tea or coffee, beer, and cola drinks. As long as their hunger is satisfied, they assume that what they are eating is good for them. So they happily stuff themselves with low-fibre, high-protein and high-fat foods – and, of course, toxins.

When they begin to suffer from indigestion, constipation, odd aches and pains and fatigue, they resort to indigestion tablets, laxatives and pain killers. If these don't bring relief, they pop a packet of multivitamin capsules into the trolley next time they go to the supermarket. When these don't have an instant effect, they dismiss "all this health talk" as rubbish and merrily continue on their toxic path.

AFTER DETOX

As you are reading this book, hopefully you have abandoned such bad habits. After your detox, you will feel in better health than you have enjoyed for years. Resolve to keep it that way. Obviously, you will now need to return to a normal diet. No matter how well you feel, do not be tempted to remain on the detox regime indefinitely. So what is a normal but healthy eating pattern?

CULTIVATING GOOD EATING HABITS

Developing good eating habits is easy. Advice is readily available. At times it seems that every newspaper and magazine in the country is concerned with healthy diets. Even supermarkets carry leaflets containing advice on how to eat for maximum health. It all comes down to just seven easy-to-keep rules.

Far left: as long as their hunger is satisfied, most people assume that what they are eating is good for them.

Below: when traditional cures for digestive problems don't have an instant effect, many who have lived a life of bad habits dismiss "all this health talk" as rubbish and merrily continue on their toxic path.

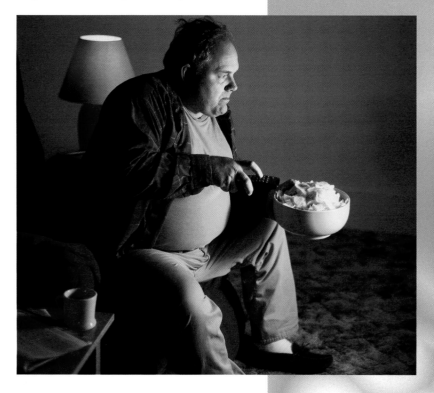

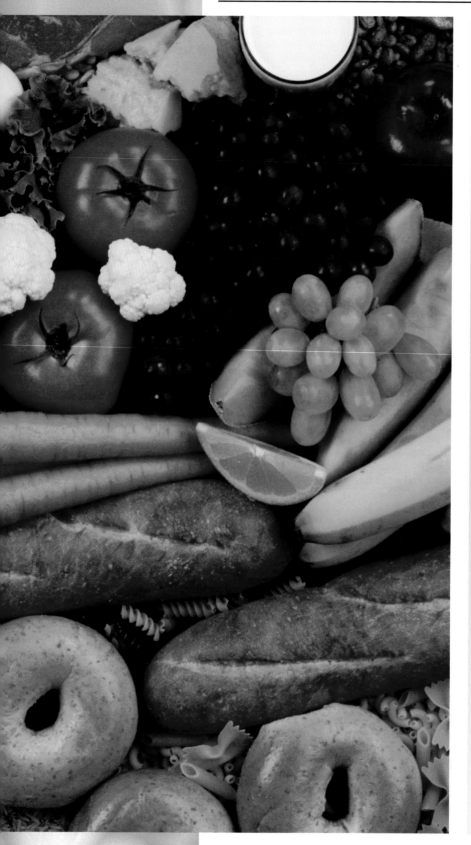

SEVEN RULES FOR HEALTHY EATING

1. *Avoid preserved, packaged or convenience food. Eat fresh food wherever possible.*

2. *Major on vegetables and fruit, raw or lightly cooked.*

3. *Maintain your fibre intake by eating wholegrain products, such as wholemeal bread.*

4. *Eat fish and poultry rather than red meat or made-up dishes such as burgers or sausages.*

5. *Cut down on your consumption of fat – but don't entirely eradicate it. Avoid saturated fats.*

6. *Drastically reduce your intake of sugar.*

7. *Eat wholemeal pasta and brown rice. When you cook potatoes, don't remove the skin.*

It isn't difficult to keep to these seven rules, if you give a little thought to how you shop and what you store in your larder, refrigerator and freezer.

The time element

For most people, the main problem is TIME. Everybody is always in a hurry. It's tempting to buy "instant meals" at the supermarket. They can be heated in the microwave while you get ready to go out. But how do these "ready meals" compare with the suggestions for healthy eating listed above?

They're packaged, so certainly not fresh.

Even vegetarian dishes are likely to contain a number of additives and, once heated, will almost certainly be over-cooked.

Not many such meals contain wholegrains of any description.

The additives and preservatives in the food can undermine the value of any fish or poultry in it. Often, the contents of these meals are "reconstituted" – that is, made up from scraps and "shaped".

Fat content is likely to be high.

Look at the list of ingredients. You're likely to find sugar listed in every packet you pick up.

Pasta or rice used is almost invariably white.

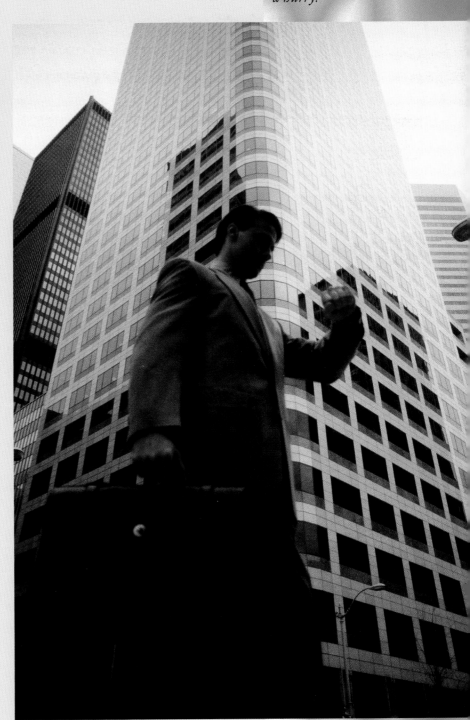

Below: the main problem for many people is time – everyone is always in a hurry.

Below: for breakfast, eat a piece of fruit and throught the day try to drink as much water as possible.

DIY INSTANT MEALS

In fact, with a little forethought, it's easy to prepare your own "instant meals" and store them in the freezer until needed. Simply check the ingredients listed on the packet of your favourite meal, and make it yourself. All the additives and preservatives will be omitted and you'll find the finished product will be considerably cheaper. The meals will also be much more satisfying and flavourful.

You'll need to shop for the food items you need, plus a supply of microwave-safe containers. After that, an evening spent in the kitchen can easily provide you with meals to last at least a couple of weeks. But do remember that the ingredients you use must comply with the seven rules.

Try healthy eating for a week. You have much to gain and nothing to lose. So what is the ideal diet for your first day?

HEALTHY EATING – DAY 1

Breakfast
A piece of fruit (apple, orange, pear or grapes.) Chew well.
A bowl of unsweetened muesli, or other "whole" cereal with a little skimmed milk.

Lunch
A jacket potato with a green salad.
A piece of fruit.

Dinner
A small portion of grilled fish or chicken with plenty of steamed vegetables or a large salad.
Fruit and/ or "live" yogurt for dessert.

Drinks
Maintain a good fluid intake throughout the day. Drink as much water as possible, plus herbal teas, diluted fruit juice or (if you're a coffee addict) a coffee substitute. You will find several on sale at your local health shop. Do they taste like coffee? Judge for yourself.

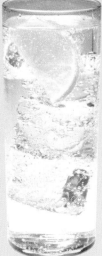

The menu given above is basic. Now I'll tell you how to make it more interesting.

VARYING YOUR DIET

Obviously, you won't want to eat the same food – or even the same type of food – every day for the rest of your life. Don't worry, that isn't necessary. Listed below are a wide variety of permissible – and delicious – foods that are guaranteed to maintain that wonderful "clean" feeling you experience immediately after your detox.

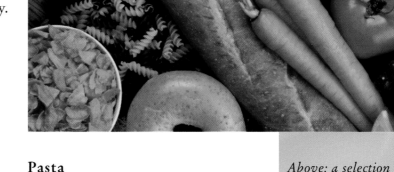

Above: a selection of food types.

Vegetables
You may eat all vegetables, but try to keep a balance between leafy and root varieties. These can be steamed or grilled. Potatoes should remain unpeeled and preferably be baked. On no account should you fry vegetables (except in a stir fry, which requires a minimum of fat) or add oily dressings.

Fruit
As with vegetables, any fruit is good for you. It all depends on your own taste and the reaction of your body. If a fruit upsets you, avoid it. Fruit is best eaten raw, but light cooking will still preserve most of the nutrients.

Meat
"Red" meat is best avoided in favour of poultry. Eat only small portions.

Fish
Any fish is preferable to meat, but "oily" varieties such as tuna, salmon and mackerel are particularly good.

Pasta
Stick with wholemeal pasta and brown rice. When making pasta sauce, avoid using minced meat. Instead, try a soya substitute.

Dairy foods
"Live" yogurt makes a delicious breakfast or dessert. Use skimmed or semi-skimmed milk sparingly and avoid full fat milk. Choose low-fat spreads in place of butter. If you're a cheese addict, drastically restrict your intakeor try the low-fat variety. Cottage cheese can often help to wean you off high-fat Cheddar, Wensleydale, etc.

Drinks
Water (again!). Diluted fruit juices. Herbal teas. Green tea. Avoid caffeinated and fizzy drinks. Use up to one pint of skimmed milk per day (this includes milk on cereals etc.).

Snacks
Dried fruits. Nuts (unsalted). Avoid chocolate and sugary sweets.

GETTING USED TO A NEW EATING PATTERN

At first, you won't be exactly over-the-moon with this new eating regime. You'll miss fried eggs and sausages and burgers etc. even though you now realise they're not good for you. You just have to take the time for your taste buds to adjust to the new sensations you are introducing. Stick with it – the end result is worth the trauma. One big bonus that you will notice as the weeks go by is that you will discover the true natural flavours of the food you eat. This can be a very pleasant surprise.

One way of dealing with "withdrawal symptoms" is to make a hobby of searching for tasty and unusual recipes. A few are listed to get you started.

Below: at first, you won't be exactly over-the-moon with this new eating regime.

Recipes

WARM VEGETABLE SALAD

Ingredients
2 oz carrots
4 oz fresh green beans
4 oz sugar snap peas
4 small potatoes (chopped into chunks)
A few cauliflower florets
1 courgette, sliced
1 clove garlic
2 fl oz extra virgin olive oil
Lemon juice
Basil, marjoram, chives to taste

Method
Steam potatoes until tender. Place in a bowl with garlic and olive oil.

Steam the other vegetables. Add to the potato mixture. Sprinkle with chopped herbs. Add lemon juice and mix.

Serve immediately on warm plates.

Serves 2/3
Obviously, any vegetables you have to hand can be prepared in this way. The recipe is highly adaptable and can be adjusted to serve any number of people.

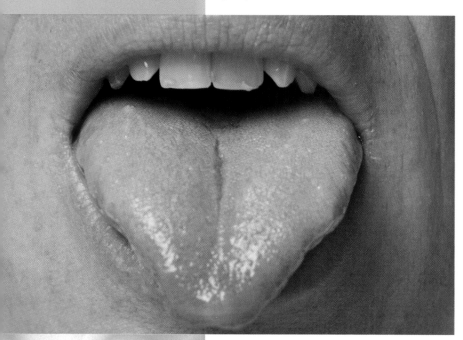

STUFFED COURGETTES

Ingredients
2 medium courgettes
4 tsp olive oil
1 small red onion
1 tsp cumin seeds
2 tomatoes
2 grated carrots

Method
Heat the oven to Gas Mark 5 (190°C/375°F). Slice the courgettes in half lengthwise and remove flesh, leaving about ¼" (6mm) in the shell. Place the sliced onion and the cumin seeds in a pan with a little water. Heat gently until the onion is softened. Add the chopped tomatoes and cook for a further two or three minutes. Add the grated carrot and the flesh from the courgettes. Cook gently for five minutes or until softened. Pile the mixture into the prepared courgette shells. Place on foil in an oven-proof dish and cook in the oven for 30–45 minutes until the shells are soft.

Serve with steamed small new potatoes.

Serves 2

APPLE SOUP

Ingredients
1 tbs sunflower oil
1 small onion, chopped
1 stick celery, chopped.
1 eating apple, cored and chopped
1½ oz plain flour
½ pint semi-skimmed milk
¼ pint chicken stock
Salt and pepper

Method
Lightly fry the onion and celery in the oil, until soft. Add the apple and cook for one or two minutes. Gradually add flour, milk, stock and seasoning. Stirring constantly, bring to the boil until the mixture is thick and smooth. Simmer for five minutes. Serve in hot bowls.

This soup can also include 1oz grated Cheddar cheese, if wished. Stir in after the mixture has thickened.

Serves 2

MARJORIE'S SOUP

Ingredients
3 large onions
1 green pepper
1 head of celery
Half a small cabbage
2 tins chopped tomatoes
1 can good quality French onion soup
1 vegetable stock cube

Method
Cut all the vegetables into small pieces. Place in a large saucepan. Add the tomatoes, soup and crumbled stock cube. Cover with water and season to taste. Add a few herbs if you wish. Simmer until all vegetables are soft. Liquidise if you prefer a smooth soup. Serve with hot crusty bread and cottage cheese as a satisfying lunch.

Sauces
These easy-to-make sauces are useful for serving with salads, pasta, etc.

Serves 2/3

SPINACH AND BASIL SAUCE

Ingredients
1 lb fresh spinach leaves
6 leaves fresh basil
1 tbs soy sauce
1 clove garlic, crushed
2 tbs semi-skimmed milk
Lemon juice
Salt and pepper to taste

Method
Thoroughly wash spinach leaves. Place crushed garlic in olive oil and fry gently for one minute. Drain spinach, place leaves on top of the garlic in the saucepan. Put the lid on the pan, turn up the heat slightly and cook until the spinach softens. Stir gently, from time to time, to ensure the garlic does not stick to the pan.

When the spinach is cooked, transfer the mixture to a blender and add the remaining ingredients. Blend to a light cream. Before serving, transfer the sauce to a saucepan and heat gently.

Be careful with the seasoning of this sauce. Too much salt will ruin it.

MUSHROOM AND THYME SAUCE

Ingredients

½ lb mushrooms
2 tbs plain flour
8 fl oz vegetable stock
1 tsp chopped thyme
1 tbs soy sauce
6 fl oz semi-skimmed milk
Olive oil
Salt and pepper

Method

Clean mushrooms and dry them. Slice and sauté in a little olive oil for five minutes. Sprinkle the flour over the mushrooms in the pan, stir well and slowly add the stock, stirring all the time. Bring to the boil, add soy sauce, and thyme and simmer gently for five minutes. Add milk, heat through gently and season. A little yeast extract may be added to this sauce, if wished, to add to the flavour.

Heat very gently after you have added the milk, or the sauce will curdle.

OVER TO YOU

As these recipes prove, a healthy diet is far from boring. Gradually, too, you will discover that home cooking need not be at all time consuming – and even if it does take slightly longer than ready meals, you will find that it is worth the time and effort you spend on it.

GO ORGANIC

Wherever possible, use organic foods. We are all aware that nowadays crops, vegetables, fruit and meat are drenched with various chemicals and preservatives. They may slightly enhance the appearance of the food, but they destroy the flavour and ensure that we increase our intake of toxins. Spend a little extra – and be sure that you're eating only the very best food available.

Below: it is worth spending a little extra to be sure you are eating the best food available.

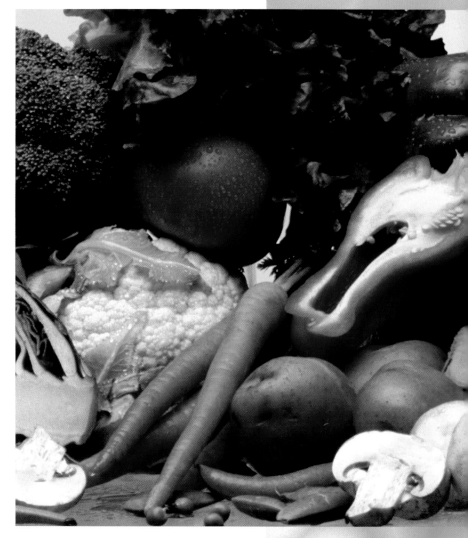

SUPPLEMENTING YOUR DIET

Below: eating a healthy diet, you should not need to supplement it.

Some nutrition experts claim that if you are eating a healthy diet, you should not need to supplement it with pills and potions. Others maintain that supplements are essential, because so much of the natural goodness of our food is destroyed by modern intensive farming methods.

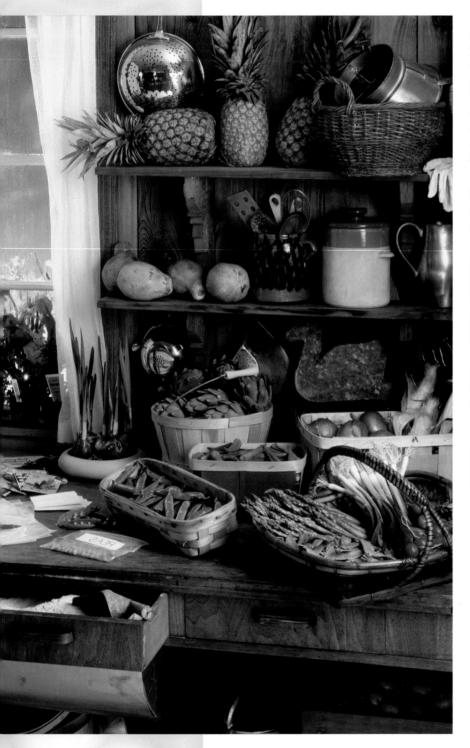

Professor Tim Lang of the Centre for Food Policy at Thames Valley University agrees, particularly insofar as minerals are concerned. A recent study showed that vegetables and fruits, in particular, have a much lower mineral content than they did even 50 years ago. In general, mineral levels are considerably reduced, as the following table shows.

Vegetables	Mineral loss
Runner beans	Almost 100% of sodium
Watercress	93% of copper
Broccoli	75% of calcium
Spinach	60% of iron
Potatoes	47% of phosphorous
Fruits	
Oranges	67% of iron
Avocado	62% of sodium
Strawberries	55% of calcium
Melon	45% of magnesium
Raspberries	39% of calcium

The vegetables and fruits listed here are not the only ones affected in this way, but they serve as a representative selection of what is happening to the nutritional values of the food we eat.

For example, the selenium levels of the soil in which they grow are drastically reduced, thanks to "acid rain", artificial fertilisers and intensive agriculture. Thus, although brazil nuts, wholemeal flour, sunflower seeds, mushrooms and a number of other foods are supposedly rich in selenium, there is no way of ensuring this. It all depends on where they are grown.

So the question must be –

To supplement or not to supplement?

The quick answer to that question is that the ubiquitous multivitamin and mineral pills stocked in supermarkets are probably sufficient for everyday use. In view of various reports such as the one mentioned above, it is probably not a good idea to rely entirely on your diet to provide the nutrition you require. On the other hand, there is no point in spending vast sums of money on supplements you don't need. Judge for yourself. If you feel fine, the combination of a healthy diet and one pill a day is probably OK for you.

However, it may be a good idea to take a course of certain supplements at any time when you're feeling stressed or have been ill or are constantly tired. But how do you know which ones to take?

Which supplement?

A number of readily available and popular supplements can be almost guaranteed to give you a boost. As they can be obtained over the counter, they are also perfectly safe. So, if you're simply feeling "under the weather", you can confidently consider:

Vitamin C
The "standard" remedy against coughs and colds and a valuable source of nutrients.

Garlic
It is called "Nature's antiseptic" and is invaluable for guarding you against infection. It also helps to maintain a healthy heart and circulation. Don't worry about the smell. There are a number of odour-free supplements on the market.

Cod liver oil/halibut liver oil
Both are rich in Vitamins A and D, which promote healthy skin, bones and teeth. The oils are particularly valuable in the winter when sunshine is noticeable by its absence.

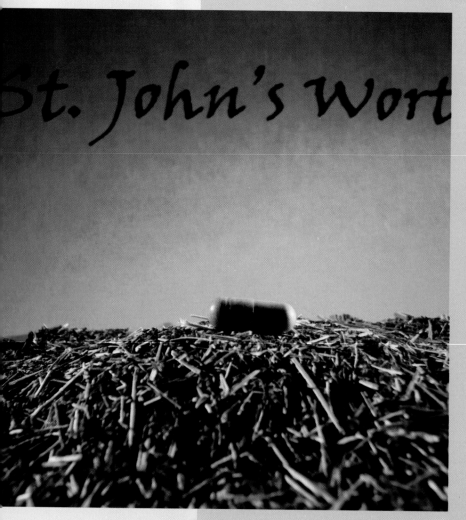

Above: St John's Wort.

Vitamin B complex

B vitamins are considered to be essential to the healthy development and functioning of the brain, nervous and digestive systems.

St John's Wort

Popularly known as "the sunshine herb", St John's Wort is famous for its depression-busting qualities and for the relief of nervous exhaustion.

NB: If you are taking anti-depressant medication, consult your doctor before taking St John's Wort.

Kava Kava

Sometimes called "the stress buster", Kava Kava is useful if you are under too much stress. It will help you to relax and unwind at the end of a trying day. It is said to promote restful sleep and may also be helpful to women during the menopause.

Selenium

Once regarded as toxic, selenium is now considered an essential trace element. In a carefully controlled dose, sometimes combined with Vitamins A, C and E, it is a vital part of the body's antioxidant enzyme defences, mopping up "free radicals".

Ginkgo Biloba

Ginkgo is thought to help to maintain the circulation of the blood to the brain and to the extremities. This stimulates brain activity and helps to maintain physical performance.

Ginseng

Ginseng helps to maintain that "get up and go" feeling. It's an adaptogen: in other words, it helps you to adapt to demanding situations and to overcome the lethargy induced by over-tiredness.

Co-enzyme Q10

This substance is found in all our body cells and its function is to help release energy from food. It can be an ideal boost if you're constantly tired, despite eating a healthy diet.

DECIDE WHAT YOU NEED.

You certainly will not need to take all these supplements, but each is extremely valuable in its own way. If you can't make up your mind which supplement is best suited to your individual needs, pop into your local health food shop. The staff will be able to advise you.

NB: On no account should you be tempted to exceed the recommended dose of any supplement. This is definitely not a case when "more" = "better".

Over-the-counter supplements are absolutely safe if taken as directed. Over-dosage can bring about uncomfortable, if not dangerous, results.

HOW LONG TO TAKE THEM

Generally speaking, you will obtain most benefit from taking a course of your selected supplement(s), rather than making them a permanent feature of your diet. Take advice from the people in your local health shop or consult a nutritionist if you are concerned about this aspect.

Alternatively, stop taking a supplement once you've used up all the pills or capsules supplied. It's easy to get more if you find that you need them.

Below: Ginkgo Biloba.

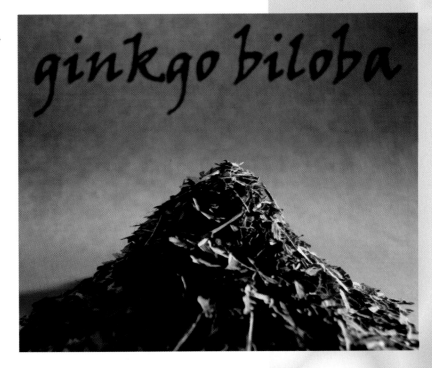

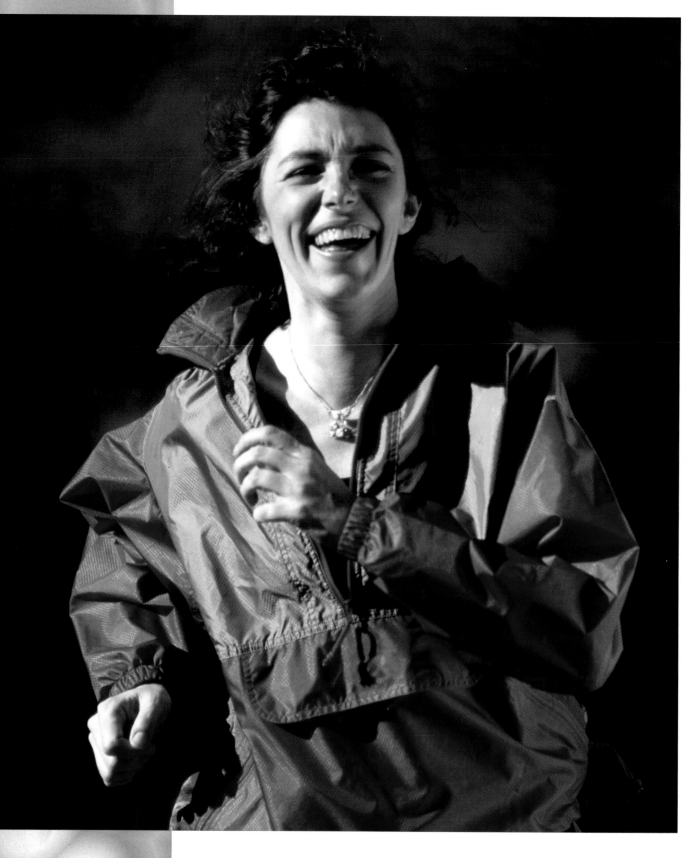

There's an old saying to the effect that we should all aim for "a healthy mind in a healthy body". That may sound stuffy. Nonetheless, it's absolutely true. However, current ideas about mental health are probably more concerned with our ability to cope with life than with the noble aspirations suggested by the adage.

SELF-ASSESSMENT QUIZ

Answer the following questions to find out how you score in this respect. Don't stop to think about your answers. Simply tick whichever response seems most natural to you.

1. What is your reaction to a disappointment?

(a) "It always happens to me."

(b) "Why do other people always get what they want?"

(c) "Maybe something better is just around the corner."

2. What is your reaction to a sudden change?

(a) "I'm scared I can't cope."

(b) "I don't want to change. Why should I?"

(c) "This could be interesting. Change is always a challenge."

3. What is your reaction when you're turned down for promotion?

(a) "I'll never get anywhere. I'm not good enough."

(b) "It's not fair."

(c) "I'll try again for the next promotion."

4. What is your reaction when a relationship breaks up?

(a) "I hate him/her."

(b) "I feel so humiliated."

(c) "I guess we weren't right for each other, after all."

5. What is your reaction when you lose your wallet?

(a) "You can't trust anybody these days."

(b) "I'm such a fool."

(c) "That will teach me to be more careful."

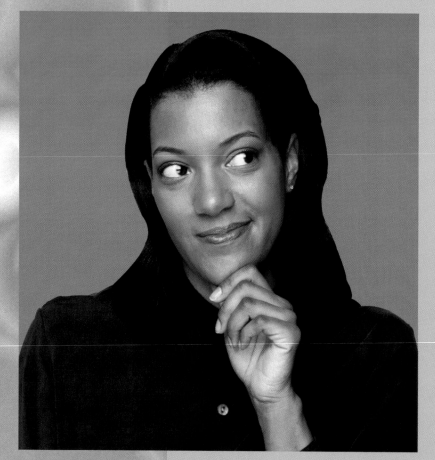

Above: how did you score?

HOW DID YOU SCORE?

The (a) and (b) answers indicate that you have problems in dealing with fairly common situations. You tend to under-value yourself or to feel resentful about other people's good fortune. The (c) answers show that you're confident of your ability to cope with most everyday events.

This quiz is designed merely to give you the opportunity to assess your mental and emotional states. It has probably never occurred to you to do this before. If your answers were mainly (a) or (b), you need to take a long look at the way you react to common situations. And even if you scored (c) on all five questions, it's highly likely that there are certain other areas in which you're less well-balanced than you thought.

Don't make matters worse by feeling guilty or resentful or disappointed about your score, whatever it is. So you didn't get all the answers right. Join the club! We all have our hang-ups. Now that you have detoxed your body, it's time to give your mind a spring clean, too.

The first step is to consider:

YOUR INTERNAL BELIEFS

"The model of human emotional disturbance" was a theory developed more than 30 years ago by Dr Albert Ellis, a clinical psychologist. He asserted that everybody has an internal belief system; in other words, we all cling to certain convictions about people and life and events. These convictions may come from our families, our peers, or from past experiences. They probably date back to our childhood and adolescence, but – even if we don't realise it – they still control our perceptions and therefore influence every aspect of our lives.

ELIMINATE THE NEGATIVE

Recent reports suggest that a large proportion of the population are adversely influenced by their internal beliefs, most of which are negative.

37% suffer from lack of self-esteem
33% suffer from guilt feelings
25% suffer from medical conditions caused by worry and anxiety

Do you come into any of these groups? Then it's time to do something about it.

Negative thoughts are every bit as toxic to your mind as a poor diet is to your body. So your first step must be to consider exactly what convictions you are feeding yourself.

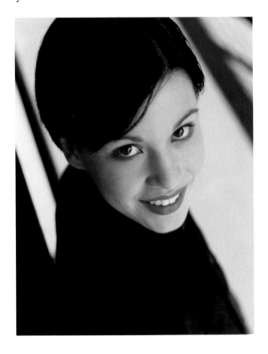

DO YOU LACK SELF-ESTEEM?

If you gave mainly (a) and (b) answers to the quiz, then you are almost certainly lacking in self-confidence. Think about it. Do you:

hate to be the centre of attention?

dread meeting new people?

find it difficult to hold a conversation?

feel that your opinion on any subject is worthless?

believe that in every way – your abilities, your appearance, your education – you are inferior to other people?

blame yourself whenever anything goes wrong?

In short, if you're the sort of person who hastily apologises when some clumsy great oaf stands on your foot – you lack self-esteem.

And many experts believe that lack of self-esteem is the basic reason why so many of us experience the problems previously listed – guilt, negative thinking, suppressed emotions, and worry.

Left: your first step must be to consider exactly what convictions you are feeding yourself.

You may like to spend a while considering exactly why you have such a low opinion of yourself. Your parents probably told you many times – as parents do – that you were "a bad girl/boy". They really meant that at that time your behaviour didn't fit in with their wishes. Your teacher, too, wasn't thinking about your self-esteem when she said, "You're so slow – you'll never get anywhere." She really meant that she was exasperated that you hadn't immediately grasped what she had just told you.

The point I'm making is that you believed all the denigrating remarks made to you when you were a child. Undoubtedly, too, the process continued in your adult life. You asked a girl for a date and she turned you down. Your boss blamed you for losing an important file (that was eventually found in his desk drawer.) And so it goes on.

What you need to remember is that most of the time people don't really mean what they say. And even if they do mean the negative comments they make to you, it doesn't necessarily follow that what they say is true. For that matter, even if the remarks were true at the time they were made – if, for example, you had lost that important file, is it sufficiently important that you should allow it

to shape the rest of your life? Winston Churchill was considered a complete dunce when he was at school – and ended up as one of the greatest prime ministers ever. When Catherine Cookson timidly submitted a story to a publisher, she was advised to take up knitting. Instead, she went on to become a successful novelist.

Look at it this way. You've received a lot of put-downs – and as the years go by, you'll undoubtedly get many more. You're not about to spend the rest of your life feeling inferior. So what can you do about these blows to your self-esteem?

IT'S TIME TO DETOX YOUR MIND

The first sections of this book concentrated on your bodily or physical health and explained how toxins can affect you. We started out by defining a toxin as "any substance that creates harmful or irritating effects in your body". For "substance" read "thought" or "idea"; for "body" read "mind". There's your definition of "mind toxins" – any thought that creates harmful or irritating effects in your mind.

Does your mind need a detox? If you're suffering from low self-esteem, the answer is a loud and definite "YES"! So let's get cracking.

GETTING STARTED

As with the body detox, your first step must be to decide on when you're going to begin. This isn't a project you can do now and again, as the fancy takes you. So as with the body detox, you'll need to make a commitment. A complete mind detox can be a lengthy process, but it's impossible to specify a time. Resolve that you will stick with the process for as long as it takes. Be assured, too, that if you enter into this wholeheartedly, you will swiftly begin to notice results.

SHOPPING LIST

You won't need to stock your cupboards with special foods for a mind detox. Obviously, you should stick with the healthy diet that (I hope) you have adopted following your body detox. The only shopping you may need to do now is to buy a large A4 notebook with lined pages. Choose a bright colour for the binding, so that you will enjoy writing in it. Ensure that you have a supply of ballpoint pens. It's extremely frustrating if your pen runs out of ink and it's the only one you have.

MAKE A LIST

Your first task in undertaking a mind detox is to try to work out where, when and how your lack of confidence originated. One way to do this is to make a list of every negative experience you can remember. Use your nice new notebook for this and realise that the task will spread over at least several days. In fact, it's a good idea to carry a small notebook with you as you go about your daily life, because memories can pop into your head at any time. Simply make a note of them and transfer them to your workbook when you get home.

When the list is finally completed, go through the events you have written down and ask yourself which of them are still having an effect on your life. Most of them will have ceased to matter, but you may well see that some – usually the most trivial incidents – are still causing problems.

Below: you won't need to stock your cupboards with special foods for a mind detox.

Below: your own uncertainty, resulting from those remarks and situations.

LIST NO 2

Make another list now – hopefully a much shorter one – of comments and events from the past that still affect you.

As you go through your list of put-downs, you'll begin to realise that most of your lack of self-esteem can be traced back to:

careless remarks made by other people;

situations that were beyond your control at the time;

your own uncertainty, resulting from those remarks and situations.

You may be surprised to discover how many of your internal beliefs have been created by unthinking remarks made many years ago. Fortunately, whether you're 15, 55 or 85, it's never too late to change your attitude and, in so doing, change your life.

THE NEXT STEP

Next time you sit down to work on this project, consider the "toxins" that are still poisoning your life. Take half a page for each one – write down brief details and then consider your current reaction. Like this:

THE GIRL WHO TURNED ME DOWN WHEN I ASKED FOR A DATE

Looking back, I can see that she wasn't all that special anyway, so I wonder why it mattered so much. Hey – wait a minute! I remember now I had a bad case of teenage acne and she laughed at me. But I'm a man now, so it can't possibly affect me. Or could it – just possibly – be the reason why I always feel awkward and ill at ease with women?

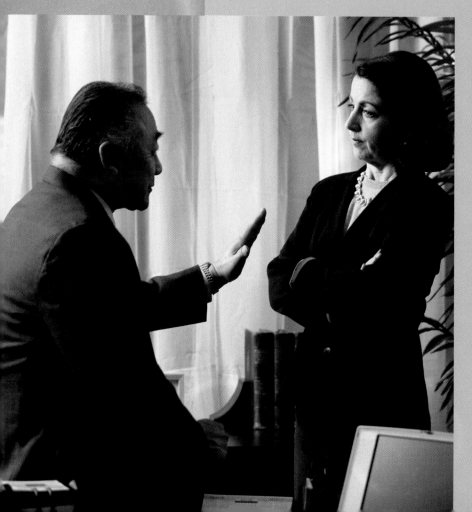

THE FILE THAT WENT MISSING

I know why it upset me so much. It was my first job and I was pretty unsure of myself, anyway. The boss was a bit of a pig, too. And to think the beastly file was in his desk drawer all the tim!. But why should it affect me now? I don't know the answer to that, but I realise that this is why I'm always nervous of authority figures, particularly men. And could it be the reason, too, I'm always saying, "I'd lose my head if it was loose"?

BE HONEST

You may find it difficult to be honest with yourself about some of the things on your list because they seem so trivial. Any time you're tempted to say, "But that's ridiculous. I'm an adult and that was a trifling event from my childhood", beware! Your reaction signifies that this particular "toxin" is one that is having a great effect on your life, even now. You're trying to devalue it merely because it is still so important and you're embarrassed about it. So grit your teeth, re-live that past experience as clearly as possible and then look at it in the context of your present life and attitudes.

Below: your reaction signifies that this particular "toxin" is one that is having a great effect on your life, even now.

WHAT COMES NEXT?

Once you feel that you've completed the recommended lists, it's time to take further action. Every now and again you're sure to remember other put-downs that still affect you, but they can be dealt with later. Right now, you are going to deal with those you have listed. There is a wide variety of techniques for doing this. Try them, one at a time, until you decide on the method you prefer.

VISUALISATION

Make yourself comfortable – in an armchair, sitting cross-legged on the floor or lying flat on a futon or yoga mat. Close your eyes and breathe deeply and regularly.

Gradually build up a mental picture of somewhere you'd like to be. This can be a real place – perhaps somewhere that you spent a superb holiday – or somewhere imaginary, like a fairy glade complete with unicorns. Don't rush this process. It's important that you should employ all your senses: "see" the beautiful scene you have created; "feel" the warmth of the sun; "smell" the flowers; "hear" the birdsong; "taste" the fresh air as you breathe in. You are creating a sanctuary to which you can escape in search of stress-free tranquillity.

Take a few minutes to enjoy this magical place. Continue to breathe deeply and regularly. Then build up another mental picture – this time of a visitor to your special place. This person is well-dressed, relaxed, happy, confident and successful.

Stay in the special place with your visitor you for as long as you wish. Then gradually come back to the present, knowing that you can repeat the experience at any time.

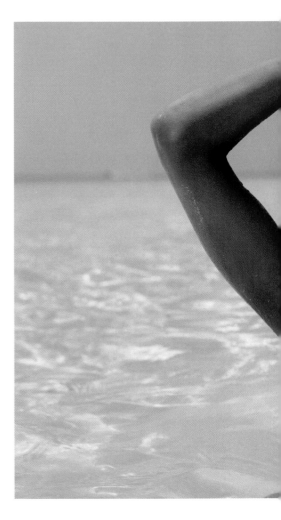

As you become more confident, you will be able to return to your sanctuary whenever you wish. In time, your visitor may hold conversations with you and even offer advice. And one day, you will make the big breakthrough – you will realise that your visitor is YOU, as you would like to be. When that happens, you can be sure that your mind detox is working. Gradually, your uncertainties and anxieties will disappear; you'll become the person you want to be – the one hidden beneath all the debris of the inner beliefs you used to hold.

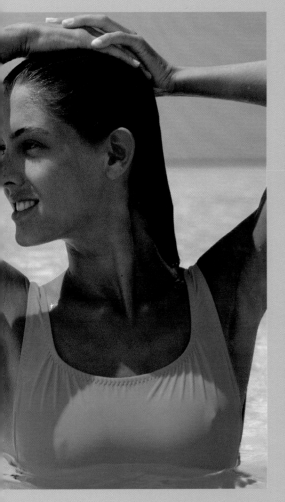

MEDITATION

This is a popular technique for relieving stress – but a lot of people have the wrong idea about it. They think that meditation involves emptying your mind – and, for the average person, this is absolutely impossible.

In fact, meditation is a process of quietening your mind, stilling the monkey chatter inside your head and finding tranquillity. Some people find this easier than others. This is what you need to do.

Settle yourself comfortably, as for the visualisation exercise. This time, though, you are advised not to lie down. If you do, you may well fall asleep. The best position for meditating is probably to sit upright in a hard-back chair, feet flat on the ground and hands loosely resting on your knees.

Close your eyes and concentrate on breathing regularly and deeply. For a few minutes, concentrate on your breath as you inhale and exhale. Then, when you feel ready, begin to concentrate on a beautiful object. For example, you could call to mind an image of a leaf. Examine it, carefully and gently, trying to keep your mind focused on the leaf and nothing else. Other thoughts will come into your head, but let them drift into your mind and out again.

Left: when visualising build up a mental picture of somewhere you'd like to be. This can be a real place – perhaps somewhere that you spent a superb holiday.

Far right: practising every day and eventually you will find that you can meditate for 20 minutes or half an hour, without problems.

Answer the following questions to find out how you score in this respect. Don't stop to think about your answers. Simply tick whichever response seems most natural to you.

1. What is your reaction to a disappointment?

(a) *"It always happens to me."*

(b) *"Why do other people always get what they want?"*

(c) *"Maybe something better is just around the corner."*

2. What is your reaction to a sudden change?

(a) *"I'm scared I can't cope."*

(b) *"I don't want to change. Why should I?"*

(c) *"This could be interesting. Change is always a challenge."*

3. What is your reaction when you're turned down for promotion?

(a) *"I'll never get anywhere. I'm not good enough."*

(b) *"It's not fair."*

(c) *"I'll try again for the next promotion."*

4. What is your reaction when a relationship breaks up?

(a) *"I hate him/her."*

(b) *"I feel so humiliated."*

(c) *"I guess we weren't right for each other, after all."*

5. What is your reaction when you lose your wallet?

(a) *"You can't trust anybody these days."*

(b) *"I'm such a fool."*

(c) *"That will teach me to be more careful."*

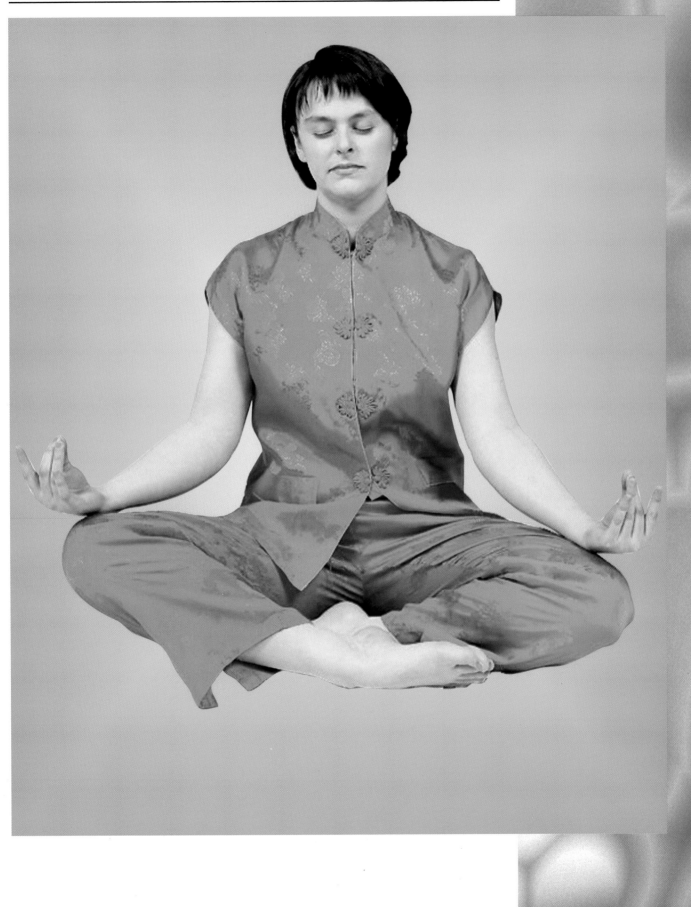

RELATIONSHIPS

Before you make changes in your life, you need to consider the other people involved. The next item on your detoxification programme is relationships. Think, for a few minutes, about all the people in your life.

You will almost certainly have relatives – and family relationships are of tremendous importance to your well-being and peace of mind.

There will be colleagues at your place of work. Since you spend most of your waking life with them, it's as well to be on good terms.

What of your employer? Do you like and respect him? If you don't, the negative feeling is likely to be mutual, so this is a situation you need to deal with quickly and firmly. Then, of course, there are your friends – what would you do without them?

And what about the dozens of people who cross your path fairly often – neighbours, the teachers at your children's school and the parents of other children, the milkman, the postman, shopkeepers, your doctor, your dentist. Until you begin to count them, you will probably not realise that your life is crowded with other people. Now is the time to consider the ways in which they affect you and whether or not you are happy with the situation.

YOUR PARTNER

Your most important relationship is probably with your partner. How do you feel about it? It's likely that you will have an instant reaction to this question – (a) I'm completely happy or (b) I wish I could get out of it.

Don't be tempted to re-think either answer. Instant reactions are usually the best, in these circumstances.

If you really do have a great relationship, there's probably no need for you to do anything more about it. Congratulations.

If, on the other hand, you really do want out, it's time to ask yourself a few more questions.

Why do I feel this way?
What is lacking in the relationship?
Which one of us has changed since the relationship began?

It may help if you write down, as clearly as possible, exactly what you feel is amiss with this relationship. At this stage, don't try to apportion blame. Just list your complaints.

Study that list for a day or two. Adjust, modify and delete as necessary. Then read it through one last time. If you still feel the same, ask your partner to read it. It's time to bring into the open all the minor and major moans and grudges.

If your partner retaliates with a list of his/her own, that's great. You have an opportunity to clear the air. It may be that some give and take and a good-tempered discussion will resolve the situation. On the other hand, the result may be an agreement that the situation is beyond repair and separation is the only alternative.

But be warned – before you undertake this particular detox exercise, you need to be absolutely sure of your own feelings. Don't compile your list just after you've had a blazing row or when you've had a bad day at the office or you're worried about the gas bill. You need to be on as even a keel as possible before you start tampering with the most important relationship in your life.

Below: your most important relationship is probably with your partner.

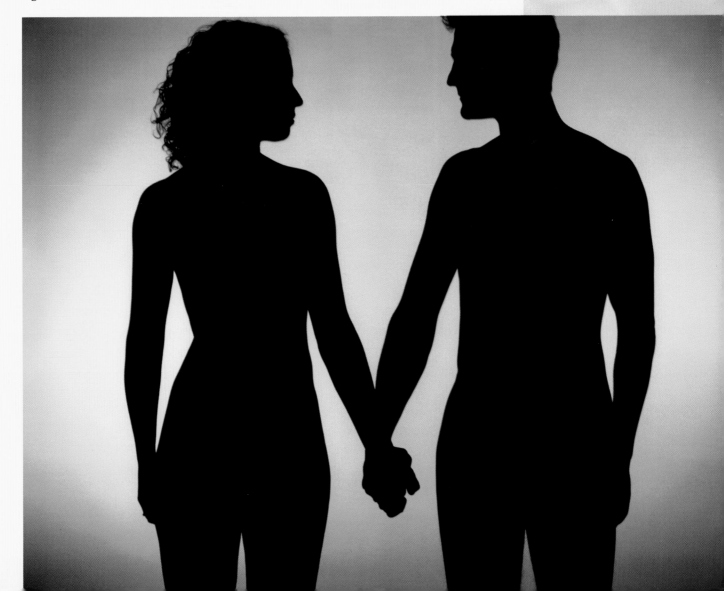

Far right: relationships have a way of working out for the best when you don't keep worrying about them.

HAPPY FAMILIES

Are you happy with your family relationships? Think about that question before you answer it.

First, consider your relationship with your parents. How often do you see them? Do you visit because you enjoy their company or because Mum and Dad expect it? Are you still living your life according to the inner beliefs they handed down to you? Or do you go your own way, but don't tell them about it?

Most adults love their parents and would hate to hurt them. At the same time, they feel a niggling resentment about certain aspects of the relationship.

"Mum expects me to tell her every detail of everything I do."

"Dad treats me like a teenager – except when he's telling me that a woman of my age should know better."

"My parents often criticise my spouse/children/friends."

"Whenever I call in, Mum has a little job for me – **just** sharpen the knives, **just** show me how to use the video. And she expects me to do everything immediately."

These are typical of the problems presented by parents – and, often, by siblings, too. What's more, they give rise to another problem. Guilt.

A friend of mine expressed it perfectly. "When I realised that I felt resentful towards my parents, I felt guilty. Then I resented the fact that they made me feel guilty – and then I felt guilty about that ... it's a vicious circle."

WHAT TO DO ABOUT IT

Try not to waste time and energy on resentment or guilt. They're toxins that can poison what should be a happy relationship. The best way to sort out this sort of problem is to be honest. If you don't explain your feelings and your needs to your family, how can you expect them to understand?

Talk to your family about the sort of relationship you would like to have with them. Ask what sort of relationship they would like to have with you. You may be surprised (and slightly put out?) to discover that your parents prefer you to call before visiting them, because they do happen to have a life of their own. Maybe your brother would like to change the regular Saturday visit to the pub because he has other things he'd rather do that night.

It's important to realise that some members of your family may be just as dissatisfied as you are with certain situations. If you have "always" done something, it can be difficult to make changes – but if you don't speak out, you run the risk of continuing on a path that doesn't really please anyone.

Plain speaking usually solves most difficulties even if, initially, there are hurt feelings and anger. Relationships have a way of working out for the best when you don't keep worrying about them.

BE FUSSY ABOUT FRIENDS

Do you find the resentment/guilt/ resentment circle also applies to some of your friends? If so, the tactics mentioned above can be helpful.

Oddly enough, you may find it more difficult to be truthful about your feelings when you're talking to friends, particularly those who have been part of your life for a long time. But you need to be choosey about the people you allow into your life. Avoid the negative types who drag you down to their level. Avoid time wasters – the people who have no aim in life and often not a thought in their heads. If you allow them to, they will waste hours of your time in idle chatter.

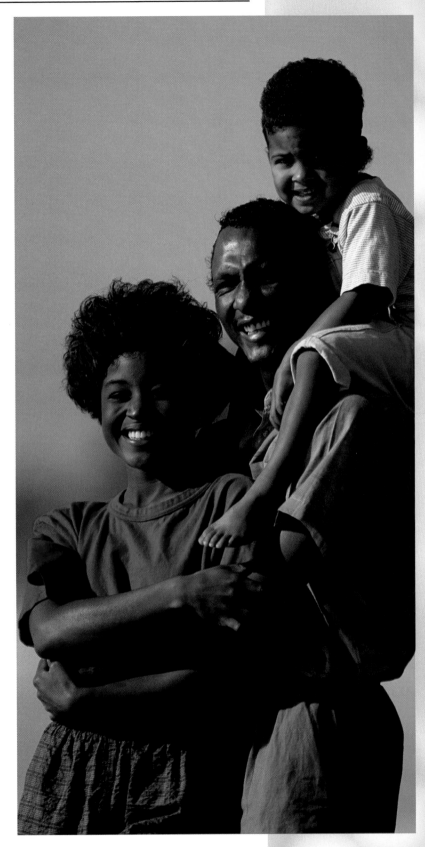

Below and far right: perhaps Mary has realised her life-long ambition to marry and have children. You have a demanding, high-powered job in finance and you enjoy every minute of it.

"WE GO BACK A LONG WAY"

Perhaps you have a friend who dates back to your childhood. She probably says proudly, "All those years – but we haven't changed a bit, have we?"

The problem is that **you** have changed a great deal. Perhaps Mary has realised her life-long ambition to marry and have children. You have a demanding, high-powered job in finance and you enjoy every minute of it.

You and Mary are both happy with your lives, but you've developed in different directions and you no longer have anything in common. As a result, your meetings are beginning to seem like a waste of time. So what can you do about it?

It is almost impossible to tell the truth. You don't want to hurt Mary's feelings. How can you possibly tell her "I don't enjoy your company any more"? This is a situation that calls for a great deal of tact – or should we be honest enough to call it subterfuge?

Begin to emphasise to Mary how very busy you are. On the next three occasions that she phones to arrange a meeting, tell her that you're snowed under with work and simply don't have the time. However, if you do make plans to meet, it's unfair to cancel at the last minute. You must keep the appointment, but ring her the day before and say you'll be an hour late or that you will have to leave earlier than usual.

If you maintain this ultra-busy attitude for a few months, you may well find that Mary gets the message and stops calling you. It's possible that she has been just as dissatisfied with the friendship as you are. On the other hand, she may go all injured – "You can't be bothered with me any more."

This is blackmail and you must not respond to it. If the injured attitude persists, be blunt and say, "I'm sorry – but we just don't seem to be on the same wavelength, any more."

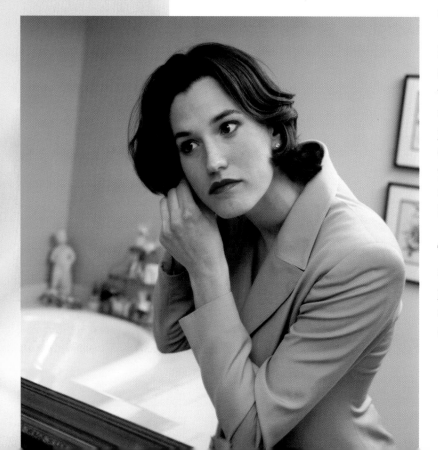

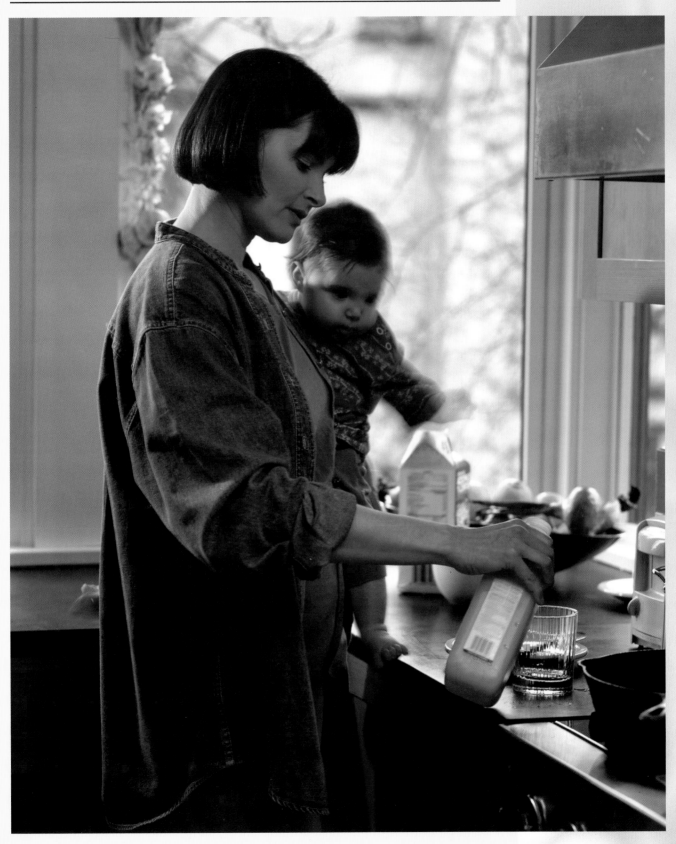

Below: a brief, firm and polite response will make your feelings clear.

THE HELPLESS TYPES

Steer clear, too, of those friends who are constantly asking you for help. Don't be too willing to support them. Most people are perfectly capable of working out their own problems, but some find it less bother to allow their friends to carry their burdens for them.

Here again it pays to be honest. The first time a friend asks you to lend her some money because she's left her purse at home, it would be churlish to refuse. The next time – if you're feeling patient – hand over the exact amount required and point out that she hasn't yet repaid the previous loan. If there is a third time, simply say, "Sorry – no." You don't have to lie and pretend that you have only sufficient money for your own fare home. A brief, firm and polite response will make your feelings clear. She'll probably be angry and injured – but does it matter? You can do without toxic friends of this sort.

BE YOUR OWN BEST FRIEND

Don't feel guilty if you follow any of the suggestions given here. When you went on a diet to detox your body, you were quite proud of your ability to stick with the project. When you detoxed your mind, you realised that it made sense to get rid of all the unhealthy ideas and thoughts you'd been harbouring. The same reasoning applies to relationships. Once you've sorted them out, you'll feel in better health, temper and spirits than ever before.

There's more to the golden rule than "love thy neighbour". The full directive is that you should "love thy neighbour **as thyself**".

This may sound selfish or strange, but why shouldn't you love yourself? You are unique. Nobody in the world is exactly like you. Be proud of that.

In your notebook, make a list of all the things you like about yourself – and don't be modest. List your talents, your virtues and what you like about the way you look. If you're honest, you'll be agreeably surprised at the length of your list.

If you really can't think of many things you like about yourself, watch your behaviour for the next day or two. Give yourself credit where it is due.

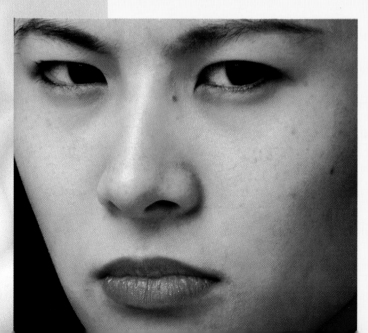

I didn't get mad when the postman delivered my mail to the house next door. We all make mistakes.

I looked after my neighbour's cat while she was on holiday.

My friend told me for the 20th time all about her new grandson and I even asked to see a photograph.

Notice the little things. Other people do, and that's why you're probably more popular than you realise.

Have faith in your own value as a human being. Of course you have faults and weaknesses, but there's no need to dwell on them or feel guilty. You are a fine person with traits and talents that confirm your worth.

MAKING NEW FRIENDS

Once you have sorted out your existing relationships, perhaps it's time to think about forming some new ones. A few good friends are better than dozens of acquaintances, but there are probably some people in your life to whom you would like to be closer.

Earlier in this section we discussed the sort of people you need to avoid. Remember this – and take your time, too, about deciding on whom you really want to draw into

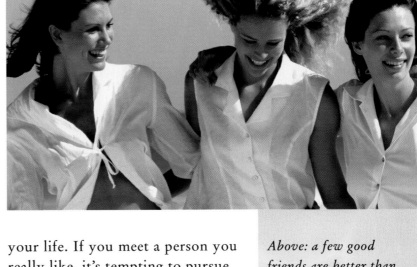

your life. If you meet a person you really like, it's tempting to pursue the acquaintance immediately. This can be dangerous. After a few more meetings you may find that you're really not on the same wavelength after all – and then you could find yourself lumbered with another toxic friend.

JOIN THE CLUB

It's a hackneyed comment, but joining a club or an evening class is one of the easiest ways to meet new people who share your interests. Don't rush into forming new relationships. Sometimes, it's a good idea to let the other person make the running at first. If this sounds stand-offish or conceited, just remember the toxic friends from whom you've freed yourself. Resolve not to repeat those mistakes – ensure that your friendship "diet" is healthy and toxin-free.

Above: a few good friends are better than dozens of acquaintances.

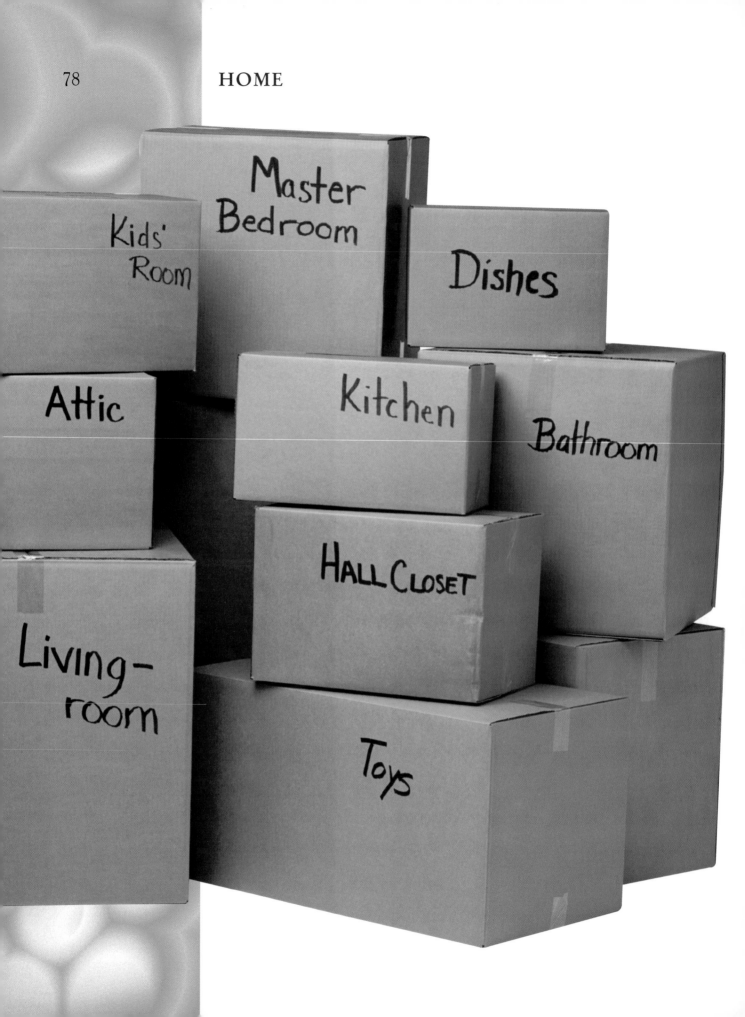

You've detoxed your body, your mind and your relationships. Now it's time to think about your home. And, as always, detoxification means getting rid of all the clutter. This is where "space clearing" comes in.

According to the ancient Chinese art of Feng Shui, clutter in your home can result in blockage of the flow of chi (life energy). This, in turn, will militate against your efforts to detox your body and other aspects of your life. Obviously, the next step in your detoxification process must be a big space-clearing exercise.

CLUTTER OR STORAGE?

Are you the sort of person who hangs on to something because "it might come in useful"? Do you keep piles of old magazines because "I want to cut out the recipes"? What about the cupboards stuffed with clothes that no longer fit you? "They're almost new and I intend to lose some weight."

According to Feng Shui, clutter and storage are two sides of the same coin. Old magazines are clutter. If you get down to cutting out the recipes and filing them neatly in a box – that's storage.

Clothes that no longer fit you are clutter – put them in bin bags and take them to the local charity shop. In fact, you'll probably find it a good idea to start your space clearing in this way. When you come back from the charity shop, you'll realise just how much space the clothes occupied in your wardrobe.

Perhaps this will inspire you to tackle your whole house. It's a massive task, but well worth the effort. Don't attempt to do the whole job in one go. To start with, it's far better to deal with only one room – and even that can be broken down to one drawer or cupboard per day, if you wish. Clearing your clutter in small "bites" ensures that you don't get over-tired or bored with the whole process.

Start your space clearing when you're feeling full of energy and enthusiasm. Then assess your willpower. You need to be strong-minded when it comes to getting rid of stuff you've hoarded for years.

If you're ready to have a go, let's begin.

Far left: clutter in your home can result in blockage of the flow of chi (life energy).

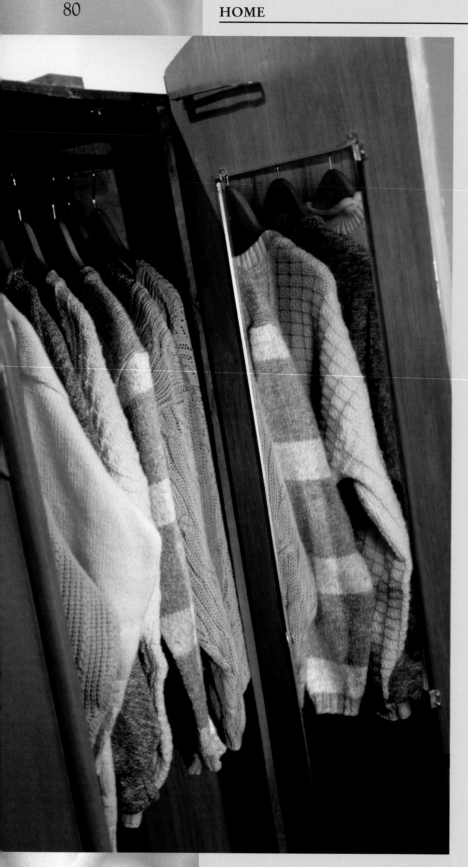

BEDROOM

Having already thrown out all those old clothes, you've made a good start. Give the interior of your wardrobe a good clean, so that it smells pleasant. Why not hang up a few lavender sachets while you're about it? Then brush your clothes and put them back in the wardrobe – you'll have plenty of space now.

Next, tackle any other cupboards in the room. Place a tray on the dressing table to hold everything you remove from the cupboards. Clean these in the same way that you did the wardrobes.

Then examine the items you've piled on the tray. Be ruthless. Throw out everything you've not used for six months or more. Dispose of medicines and toiletries past their sell-by date. At all costs, avoid the "it may come in useful" syndrome. Throw all the junk into a plastic bin bag, then put away the remaining items. You'll probably find that you now have at least one empty cupboard.

Drawers come next. Deal with them in the same way. Throw out old hair brushes and combs – why on earth would you need four of each? That dark plum lipstick didn't suit you – and it never will, even if it is a very expensive brand. This applies, too, to perfume you no longer like. In short – consign to the plastic bin bag absolutely every little item that you are not going to use tomorrow or the next day.

SECOND THOUGHTS

Jewellery is absolutely the only item on which you are allowed second thoughts. Costume jewellery, bought for one very special occasion, can be dumped. That goes, too, for things like the plastic beads worn with a long-forgotten summer dress. Think again, though, when it comes to gold or silver or Granny's string of pearls. You probably won't wear them, anyway, so take them to a jeweller for valuation. Throwing away anything of real value isn't ruthless – it's plain stupid.

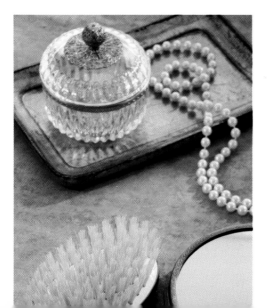

DUST TRAPS

Once you've cleared out every wardrobe, cupboard, drawer and shelf in your bedroom, you may like to glance at the various ornaments you have on display. Do they really add anything to the room or are they merely dust traps? You need the clock beside your bed, of course – but what about the books for your bedtime reading? Now that you have so much more space, the current favourite can be popped into the drawer of your bedside cabinet. Put the others into your bookcase until you're ready to start reading them.

What about the family photographs? Is it essential to have so many? Couldn't you get a "family group" – or even display a picture of just one person each week?

One beautiful, peaceful picture on the wall is fine – do you really need more? And what about mirrors? According to Feng Shui you should not have a mirror placed so that you and your partner can see yourselves in it when you are in bed.

Look at your lampshades. Are they perhaps a bit too fussy? Or are they discoloured and dusty? You may like to replace them with shades in a simple, more elegant style.

Far left: give the interior of your wardrobe a good clean.

Below: jewellery is absolutely the only item on which you are allowed second thoughts.

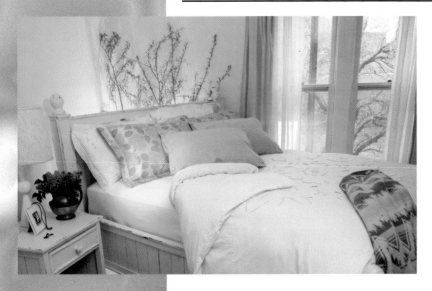

Above: glance around your spacious, tidy, airy room you'll feel it was time well spent.

Curtains, next. Do you need a Venetian blind **and** velvet curtains? Is it essential to have voile hangings **as well as** satin drapes? Why not treat yourself to new window dressings – something simple and easily cleaned?

If you have fitted carpets, you don't need bedside rugs, too. If you have laminate flooring, why not replace your thick, heavy rugs with thin washable ones?

Having read all these suggestions, you'll understand why space clearing takes a long while. But when you glance around your spacious, tidy, airy room you'll feel it was time well spent.

Indulge yourself by hanging a little set of windchimes in the window. Their delicate sound will soothe you to sleep at night and rouse you pleasantly in the morning. What's more, they'll guard you against negative chi.

LIVING ROOM

By the time you've detoxed your bedroom, you'll probably be all set to start on space clearing your living room, too. Don't rush it. If you're tired, your efforts will be less productive – and then you'll be disappointed and tempted to abandon the whole idea. Having cleared the bedroom, give yourself a couple of days off before you start on the lounge.

FAMILY OPPOSITION

Follow the same routine as you used for the bedroom. You may well find even more clutter in the living room – and will probably meet strong opposition from your family when you start clearing it out.

There's no point in arguing. If your teenager insists that he can't possibly part with even one of his CDs, and your partner vows that his stamp collection is vital to his enjoyment of life, you need to use subterfuge. Quietly move the CDs to the teenager's bedroom; that's where his player is, anyway. Soften the blow by providing a stylish new CD rack.

TACT OR SUBTERFUGE?

Carefully – **very** carefully – gather together all the odd stamps and packets littering the floor and coffee table beside your partner's armchair.

And this time, you must strongly resist the urge to dump them in the plastic bin bag. Instead, put them in a large, attractive wooden box. Then buy him a couple of classy stamp albums, provide him with a bookcase deep enough to hold them and a small table for working on. Don't forget the stamp hinges, of course, and a pair of tweezers – they can be stored in the aforementioned box. When he wants to know what's happening, you simply smile sweetly and explain that his collection needs to be valued and cared for. He'll be puzzled, of course, but pleased that you appreciate the value of his hobby.

A FAMILY ROOM

Having coped with the opposition, you can go ahead with your detoxing project. When dealing with a lounge, though, you must remember that it is essentially a family room. You are free to dispose of any of your own possessions that you no longer want or need. If you begin a wholesale clearance of family treasures, you're just asking for trouble. Your only hope of even limited success is to proceed quietly, cautiously and tactfully.

The first step is to have a grand tidy up. Clean all the shelves, cupboards and drawers as before. Then sort out the clutter and allocate it to the person who owns it. Fortunately, most of the children's stuff can be stored in their own rooms. You'll need to be persistent and patient about this. Every time a video or a skateboard is abandoned in the living room, take it back upstairs. You can at least hope that eventually the kids will get the message.

Below: you can at least hope that eventually the kids will get the message.

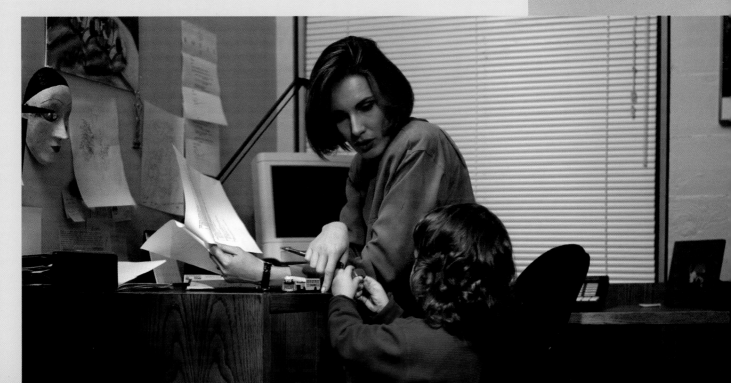

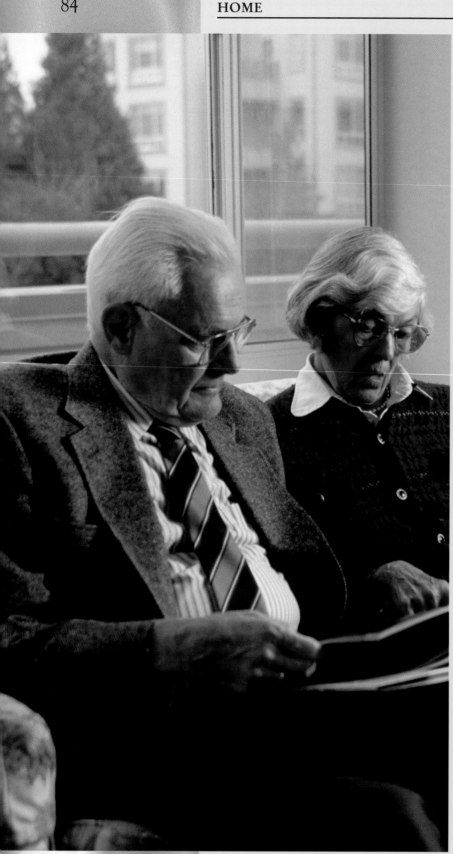

TERRITORIAL CLAIMS

So far as the adults in the family are concerned, you need to provide each one with storage space – a place where their belongings will be readily to hand. Grandad's detective stories can have one special shelf in the bookcase. Grandma's embroidery can be stored in a drawer. Explain this to them, but be careful to emphasise that the changes are for their convenience, not yours.

When they leave their belongings on the floor or behind the sofa – as they will – simply return their property to its appointed place. Adults are likely to be much more co-operative than the children. In fact, in no time at all they'll be getting highly possessive about their own storage area. People, like cats, are territorial animals.

Meanwhile, of course, you have been quietly disposing of all sorts of rubbish – though you may have to endure the hideous vase your partner's aunt gave as a wedding present or the bowl of boiled sweets Grandad likes to have at hand when he's reading.

Don't feel disheartened if at first you're less successful with detoxing the living room than you were with the bedroom. Do your best right now, but realise that this will be a long drawn-out process. You will have to do most things quietly and gradually. However, as with the bedroom, the end result will be worth all the hassle.

KITCHEN

Your kitchen will probably be much easier to detox than your living room. However, this room presents certain problems of its own, so you would be well advised to tackle it "in penny numbers". For example, you can clear and clean the cutlery drawer while you're waiting for the coffee to finish percolating and sort out the broom cupboard while the iron is heating up.

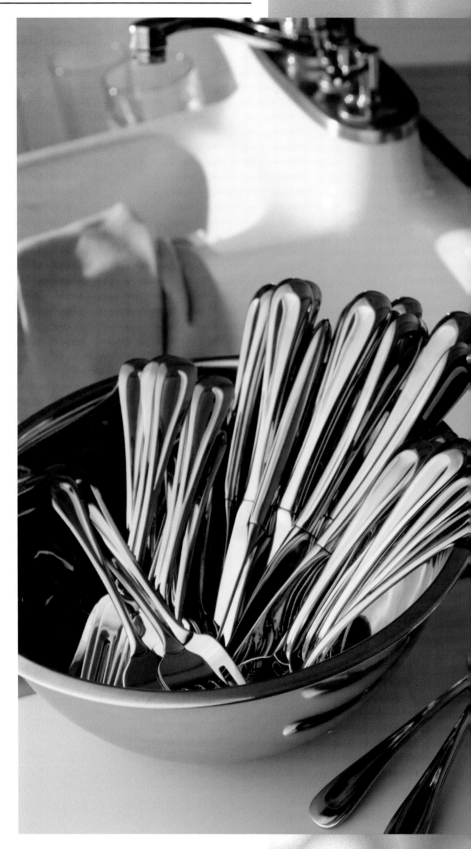

Below: you'll find all sorts of things tucked away and forgotten.

DRAWERS AND CUPBOARDS

First deal with the drawers. This won't take long. Most people tend to use kitchen drawers as a haven for things that "may come in useful" – plastic carrier bags, odd pieces of kitchen foil, the end of a candle. Your best plan is to empty the drawer straight into the rubbish bin. Then all you need to do is clean and replace it.

Cupboards come next. Deep ones are a particular hazard, because items that are seldom used get pushed to the back and forgotten. You'll probably find gunged-up sauce bottles, tins that are beginning to

rust, packets that are leaking their contents and all sorts of other horrors. Don't waste time on feeling guilty. Simply heave the lot. Put aside the items in constant use until you've cleaned the cupboards.

This may take longer than usual. Add a little disinfectant to a bowl of hot soapy water and scrub every inch of each interior. While it's drying, wipe over the tins and bottles you intend to return to the cupboard, and check on any packet goods.

As always, you'll find that you have more storage space than you realised. So much more, in fact, that you'll be able to store in cupboards some of the things currently cluttering up the working surfaces in the kitchen.

EQUIPMENT

Your next job is to clean the cooker and the microwave. Then tackle the refrigerator and the freezer. Yet again, you'll find all sorts of things tucked away and forgotten. In order to keep your kitchen immaculate and guard against a build-up of toxins, you need to make two resolutions.

Restrict your shopping list to items you really need.
Check pantry, refrigerator and freezer on a weekly basis, so that you use everything stored before it reaches its sell-by date.

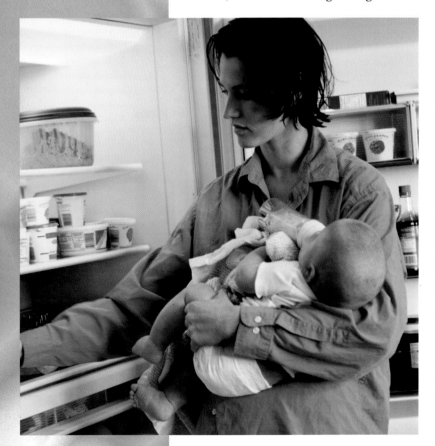

BATHROOM

This is the easiest room of all to detoxify. Follow the usual routine. If possible, take down your bathroom cabinet so that you can clean it properly, inside and out. Use disinfectant in hot soapy water, as you did with the kitchen cupboards. Scrub the loo, the bath and the wash basin. Stand the loo brush in a strong disinfectant solution; better still, buy a new one. Clean the windows and the mirrors. Launder the shower curtain and the bathroom rugs. Sort out the contents of the bathroom cabinet. You'll probably need to dispose of most of them.

After the onslaught, your bathroom will be absolutely sparkling. Keep it that way with daily attention and a weekly spring-clean. It doesn't take long and is worth the effort.

THE REST OF THE HOUSE

Halls and stairways are particularly important in the Feng Shui philosophy because the all-important chi flows along them. Try to avoid having hooks or a hall-stand in the hall. Visitors' coats can be hung in a bedroom. You must also sternly resist your family's tendency to throw their coats over the banisters as they enter the house. Ensure that stairs and passages are brightly lit and that carpets and rugs are kept in good repair. You may like to hang windchimes in the hall. According to Feng Shui, they control the flow of chi and deter evil spirits.

THE FRONT DOOR

All that remains to do now is to ensure that your front door is in good repair, paintwork immaculate, glass shining and metalwork well-polished. Not only does this create a good impression for your visitors, it will give your spirits a lift as you walk into your beautifully detoxed house. You can relax now in the satisfaction of a job well done.

Below: try to avoid having hooks or a hall-stand in the hall.

Below left: after the onslaught, your bathroom will be absolutely sparkling.

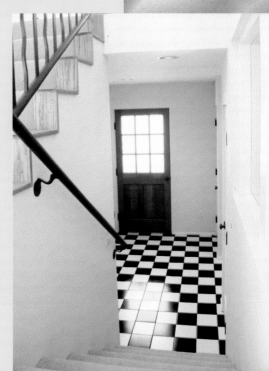

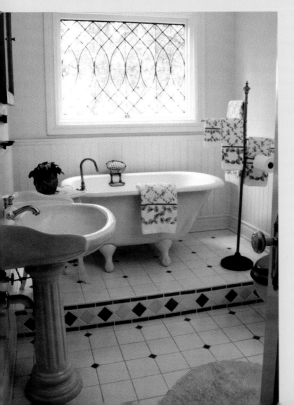

*Below: don't forget
the importance of
water. Drink at least
two litres of filtered
water every day.*

HELPING HANDS

Now that your detoxification project has been completed, you will want to maintain the good feelings it has produced. There is a variety of ways to do this.

PHYSICAL AIDS

Don't forget the importance of **water**. Drink at least two litres of filtered water every day.

Remember the soothing qualities of a warm, scented **bath**.

Bathe in **Epsom salts** to expel toxins through the skin. Add 100 gm of sea salt and 225 gm Epsom salts to a hot bath. Soak for about 15 minutes, then dry yourself quickly and get into a warm bed.

Dry skin brushing helps to sweep away all the toxins expelled through the skin during your body detox. It also improves the circulation of blood and lymph.

Using a loofah or a rough flannel, start brushing at your feet and work up towards your heart in long, firm strokes. Gradually brush the whole of your body, remembering always to move **towards** your heart and not away from it. Use gentle circular strokes in a clockwise direction when brushing your stomach.

Follow the skin brushing with your usual bath or shower.

Colonic irrigation helps to flush away the accumulation of toxins in the colon and can be extremely helpful during a detox programme. If you're uncertain about using this method, consult your health practitioner before making an appointment with a colonic therapist.

Massage, aromatherapy and saunas are all delightfully relaxing experiences that aid the release of toxins from the body.

Practise **correct breathing** until it becomes natural to you.

Remember the importance of exercise. If time is your enemy, a short stretching session or a brisk walk is better than no **exercise** at all.

Get into the habit of eating a **healthy diet**. It doesn't need to be boring – and, of course, you can allow yourself the occasional indulgence without ill effects.

Make sure, though, that the indulgence is **only** occasional and that it doesn't go too far. Eating two small squares of chocolate is an indulgence. Consuming a 250 gm bar is a binge.

Use **organic foods** whenever possible. They may be expensive, but you can't put a price on good health.

Supplements can give a useful boost to your detox efforts, but they are not intended to replace a healthy diet.

MAINTAINING A HEALTHY MIND

Start reading **self-help/personal development books**, some of which are recommended in the Appendix.

Try to **meditate** every day.

It's a good idea to **write in your workbook** every evening. This helps to clear from your mind any niggling irritations or worries you may have.

Affirmations can be repeated mentally anywhere and at any time. If you combine them with **visualisation,** you increase their effectiveness.

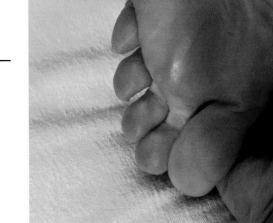

Make a habit of trying to **learn something new**. Classes and courses on any subject that interests you will keep your mind active and widen your horizons. Even reading a dictionary and learning just one new word a day keeps your mind supple. Games like Scrabble and Trivial Pursuit will keep your brain active, yet be relaxing at the same time.

Above: massage, aromatherapy and saunas are all delightfully relaxing experiences that aid the release of toxins from the body.

Below: light a scented candle in the room you are detoxing.

FORMING GOOD RELATIONSHIPS

Try not to **criticise** other people, even in your thoughts. You have no right to pass judgement on them unless their actions adversely affect you.

Conversely, try not to **resent criticism** from other people. They have a right to their opinions, but there is no need for you to accept them.

Have the courage to **be honest** about your feelings. It's possible to disagree with someone without being unpleasant.

Recognise that **relationships change**, for a variety of reasons, and there is no need to apportion blame. Accept that certain friendships may have served their purpose and are no longer viable.

Support your family and friends in any way possible, but **don't become a doormat**. Most people are capable of sorting out their own problems.

Make a habit of **congratulating yourself** when you deserve it.

Remember that **meeting new people** can often introduce fresh ideas and different dimensions to your life.

ENHANCING YOUR SURROUNDINGS

Space clearing is an ideal way to re-discover the charms of your home. Most houses don't suffer from lack of storage space. It is the inefficient use of storage that is the real problem.

Light a scented candle in the room you are detoxing. According to Feng Shui, this will get rid of stagnant chi.

Another Feng Shui method is to **clap out** each room when you have cleaned it. Stand in each corner of the room in turn. Raise your hands and clap briskly, three times, lowering your arms as you do so. Continue until you have clapped out each corner in the room. This routine is said to remove trapped energies and clear the room.

Remember that most of the cleaning products now available from supermarkets contain chemicals that can create toxins. Instead, you may like to use some of the natural cleansers listed below.

NATURAL CLEANERS

Equal quantities of white distilled vinegar and water in a spray bottle can be used for cleaning mirrors, windows and tiles.

Use a cut lemon and salt to remove limescale from an enamel bath.

Disinfect loos and sinks with tea tree essential oil.

Lemon juice can be used to clean tarnished metal.

Clean stained dishes and chopping boards by scrubbing them with salt. Equal parts of vinegar and water will remove limescale from kettles. Bring to the boil then switch off and leave overnight. In the morning, empty the kettle and rinse well. Fill with water, boil and empty again before use.

Raw potato slices will remove marks from carpets if left in place overnight.

Look in your supermarket for eco-friendly cleaning products.

HOUSE PLANTS

Use house plants to decorate and purify the air in your home. These are particularly useful in the kitchen, near to the television set and adjacent to computers.

According to NASA, the following are the Top Ten of the plant world:

Areca palm
Lady palm
Spider plant
Peace lily
Bamboo

Rubber plant
Ivy
Gerbera
Chrysanthemum
Fig plant

Feng Shui experts advise you to keep a "money plant" – (*crassula argentea*) – in your office to boost your income. The theory is that all the time the plant thrives, so will your finances.

FRESH AIR

Ensure that you air your home thoroughly every day, even in winter. Get into the habit of opening all doors and windows for 10 minutes at least twice a day. For best results, open them all at the same time.

Have all gas appliances regularly serviced.

Use an ioniser in your living room, particularly if there is a smoker in the house.

Burn aromatherapy oils instead of using chemical air fresheners.

Set your heating thermostat just one degree lower than usual. No-one will notice, you'll save on your heating bills and your home will be less stuffy.

Below: ivy, one of the top ten in the plant world.

MEET THE NEW YOU

You've reached the end of this book and you've faithfully carried out the various programmes. How do you feel?

My guess is that when you looked in the mirror this morning you were bright-eyed and bushy-tailed, full of the joy of living and eager to begin a new day.

Probably you find it difficult to remember how weary, lethargic and bored you were when you started reading. Your physical and mental health have improved beyond all recognition. Stress no longer troubles you. You're thinking more clearly – and probably aiming for promotion at work. You enjoy relaxed and fulfilling relationships with your family and friends, old and new. You're justifiably happy with your beautiful home and delight in lots of visitors. Your detoxification venture has succeeded beyond your wildest dreams and your life has changed completely.

So – is that the end of the story? I hope not. If you are to maintain – and improve – your current happy situation, you have more work to do.

WHAT HAPPENS NEXT?

A detox is not a once-in-a-lifetime event. On the contrary. You should make a habit of detoxing your body, mind, relationships and home at regular intervals. However, none of the programmes will be as difficult or time-consuming as they were at first.

If you work out a healthy diet and stick to it, you'll find a weekend detox once every three months should keep you sparkling. Better still, why not a one-day detox once a month?

You can use your workbook to detox your mind and your relationships whenever you feel like it. Why not deal immediately with any minor crisis that may crop up? The secret lies in not permitting these trivial upsets to fester and assume huge proportions.

As for your home, my guess is that you and your family will be so happy with its smart new appearance and tranquil orderly atmosphere that it will be no problem to keep it that way.

You're healthy, and you're happy with every aspect of your life. **Meet the new you!**

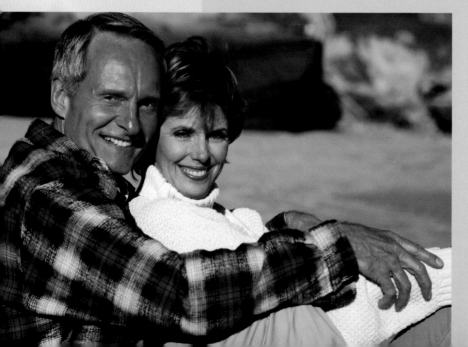

APPENDIX

FURTHER READING

THE DETOX MANUAL
Suzannah Olivier (Pocket Books –
Simon & Schuster)

BODY TONIC
Leon Chaitow (Gaia Books)

10 DAY CLEAN-UP PLAN
Leslie Keaton (Ebury Press)

MIND DETOX
Deborah Marshall-Warren
(Thorsons)

TOTAL DETOX
Jane Scrivner (Piatkus)

SPIRIT OF THE HOME
Jane Alexander (Thorsons)

PRACTICAL FENG SHUI
Richard Craze (New Life Library,
Select Editions)

BE YOUR OWN LIFE COACH
Fiona Harrold (Hodder &
Stoughton)

THE SEVEN HABITS OF
HIGHLY EFFECTIVE PEOPLE
Stephen R. Covey (Simon &
Schuster)

PURE BLISS
Gill Edwards (Piatkus)

THE POWER IS WITHIN YOU
Louise Hay (Eden Grove Editions)

USEFUL ADDRESSES

Colonic International Association
16 Englands Lane
London NW3 4TG

The School of Feng Shui
2 Cherry Orchard
Shipston-on-Stour
Warwickshire CV36 4QR

Transcendental Meditation
Freepost
London. SW1P 4YY

INDEX

INDEX

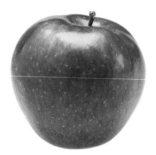